# Fasting

## The Powerful Method to Losing Weight & Improving Your Health

By:
Zilker Press

**ISBN:** 978-1-951791-60-5

# Table of Contents

Whether in the context of a broad consensus among otherwise very different and diverse religious traditions, or in the context of an emerging consensus in the modern world among medical professionals, one of the few things on which these communities appear to agree is on the usefulness and wisdom of appropriate fasting. Although ancient religious traditions such as Christianity, Judaism, Islam, Hinduism and Buddhism advocate fasting primarily for spiritual reasons, medical professionals in the contemporary world have discovered that fasting, when conducted through appropriate protocols, can yield physical health benefits such as lowering of blood pressure, weight loss and lowering of cholesterol (in many cases, of course, even many of the ancients were quite aware of the physical health benefits of fasting).

The forms and methods of fasting are as diverse as the kinds of food available to eat! There are a few primary different forms of fasting, and some of these have various protocols by which they can be carried out. For example, so-called "intermittent fasting" is a kind of umbrella term for methods of fasting that involve cycling between fasting and non-fasting at specified intervals, rather than foregoing food consumption altogether.

Although many of these protocols are structured with some degree of precision, it is possible to engage in intermittent fasting through spontaneous meal skipping. Put simply, you may want to fast simply by skipping meals whenever you feel like it. The body is quite resilient, having evolved to cope with the possibility of long periods of famine, so missing the occasional meal or two from time to time is not something that will have harmful consequences as long as you are maintaining a healthy lifestyle in other respects.

Although humans (at least in wealthier countries) no longer anticipate extended periods of little or no food, this is a reality much of the animal kingdom must still strive with. For example, wolf packs of the Northern Rocky Mountains in the United States are only treated to a sumptuous banquet of bison, deer or elk only once every couple of weeks. This means that they depend for their lives on the metabolic switch that wealthier humans can mobilize simply for the purpose of losing weight; a process that requires the ability to quickly shift their metabolism from fat storage to fat mobilization for energy by means of fatty acid β-oxidation (Anton et al., 2018). Through these physical mechanisms, they are able to store energy as lipids in fat depots where food is readily present and to then switch into "famine mode" using ketones as energy when food is unavailable. This may be why the body and the brain function at a higher capacity when using ketones as energy during periods of fasting; because we evolved in circumstances in which such preferential energy consumption was necessary for survival, and this is still true for many animals today (Anton et al., 2018).

Early humans experienced much the same reality, and many scientists believe that the superior cognitive complexity of humans emerged as an evolutionary adaptation that allowed us to construct the kinds of tools necessary to feed ourselves. Although superior brain function in wolves allows them to construct a proper "strategy" to hunt down food, humans would develop the ability to construct physical instruments as extensions of our bodies to not only hunt food, but domesticate animals, discover sophisticated methods of storing food that had been acquired, and engage in agricultural practices that could ensure the presence of food when hunting was either impossible, undesirable or unnecessary (Anton et al., 2018).

## Can Intermittent Fasting Fight Inflammation?

While inflammation is necessary to fight infection in the body, too much inflammation can cause health problems. One of the likely reasons for the onset of higher levels of dangerous inflammation in the modern world has to do with what we mentioned earlier about humans having evolved to endure periods of famine, with the modern human consuming far too much food, too often. Recent research suggests that intermittent fasting reduces inflammation; a culprit linked with an innumerably large list of serious chronic health problems. The hypothesized reason for this has to do with a decrease in monocytes, a type of cell found in the blood that causes inflammation. During their experimentation, these researchers found that monocytes in mice and humans were less inflammatory than those who were not participating in intermittent fasting. One of the researchers suggested that eating only between 11 a.m. and 7 p.m., a method more consistent with our natural circadian rhythms, might be a key to reducing the inflammation associated with overeating (Berger, 2019).

Time-restricted eating in particular, one of the researchers said, appears to improve overall gut health and microbiota. Far from affecting only the gut, these conditions affect the health of the entire body. The human participants of one study were forbidden from eating between 12pm and 3pm on the first day of the study. Those who participated in this protocol exhibited far fewer numbers of monocytes in their blood. Inflammatory bowel disease (IBD), a category of serious disease that includes Crohn's disease and ulcerative colitis, has also shown to be responsive to intermittent fasting. These diseases can cause serious damage to the lining of the bowel leading to diarrhea, weight loss, bloody stool and stomach pain. Although the causes of these diseases are unknown, they appear to be related to immune system dysfunction and abnormalities in gut microbes.

Although IBD is not caused by diet, modifications in food consumption have shown to be effective in mitigating these symptoms. One study subjected mice with inflamed bowels to a fasting-mimicking diet for 4 days which provided about half of the calories of the regular diet, another was given only water for 2 days, and another was given an ordinary diet. The group of mice who were given the fasting-mimicking diet showed improvement in their symptoms, including a return of average length to their colon, suggesting that its tissue had been regenerating. This group also exhibited enhanced growth of beneficial bacteria in the guts of the mice. The mice who had been given only water also exhibited some improvement in symptoms. Similar results were demonstrated in groups of humans who were subjected to similar protocols.

Indeed, there are quite a few studies that suggest that intermittent fasting might help with quite a few inflammatory diseases, providing some helpful, reciprocally reinforcing evidence that intermittent fasting does lower inflammation overall. In one case, a small pilot study found evidence that suggests that a 24-hour fast could inhibit a cellular pathway that contributes to asthma symptoms. Investigator Michael Sack, an M.D. and a Ph.D. is interested in how dietary interventions affect a defense system mobilized by the body known as the NLRP3 inflammasome. While the purpose of this system is to respond to threats by causing cells to release cytokines as a means of producing infection-fighting inflammation, individuals with asthma and other inflammatory diseases produce too much inflammation, as the inflammasome releases these chemicals even when they are not necessary (Jauregui, 2016).

Dr. Sack expresses concern that recent asthma research tended to exclude the inflammasome when speaking of the immune system, and evidence has only recently surfaced that the inflammasome plays a role in the inflammation symptoms generated by asthma. He conducted an experiment in which he had 18 participants fast for 24 hours, during which they consumed only water, and then gave blood samples to determine lung function. After this, they were given a meal to end their

4

fast and then given another blood draw and lung test two and a half hours later. Those who had not eaten for 24 hours showed lower levels of inflammatory cytokines associated with inflammation activity and also showed lower levels of activity in genes related to NLRP3 genes that contribute to this inflammation activity.

Evidence has also surfaced that other diseases, some having to do with immune system dysfunction, such as lupus and multiple sclerosis, might be responsive to certain fasting protocols. Research on both mice and humans has demonstrated that calorie-restricted diet was successful in reversing symptoms of multiple sclerosis and the research team that has conducted this research expressed their decision to move on with larger protocols. According to lead researcher Valter Longo from the University of South California, the fasting-mimicking diet they experimented with caused the production of cortisone that killed a larger number of autoimmune cells. He and his team developed a fast-mimicking diet that functions by cutting the number of calories consumed for 3.5 days out of 7. Earlier research that he and his team had conducted on fasting had suggested it had anti-aging effects as well (Rangan, et. al, 2019).

Mice were placed on a fasting-mimicking diet for three weeks, totaling 9 days of fasting out of 21. Relative to the control group, the mice who had been fasting reduced disease symptoms by an astonishing 20 percent. After the fasting-mimicking diet had killed the bad immune cells, the mice had returned to their ordinary diet, which saw the production of good immune cells and also myelin-producing cells, causing many of the mice to reach a state free of any disease. The study that involved human research subjects totaled 60 participants with multiple sclerosis, who either endured a fast-mimicking diet for a week followed by 6 months of a Mediterranean diet, six months of a high-fat diet or six months of a normal diet. Those who fasted and then went on a Mediterranean diet saw major improvements in both physical and mental health compared with the control group, which did not exhibit such improvement (Rangan et. al, 2019).

## Can Intermittent Fasting Help Seizures?

Some research has even begun to surface suggesting that fasting may decrease the frequency of seizures in individuals predisposed to epilepsy by calming overexcited neurons in the brain. Dr. Pejmun Haghighi, author of one study, found evidence that intermittent fasting may impact synaptic activity, which is the process in which signaling molecules known as neurotransmitters are released between neurons, altering neuronal activity. These neurotransmitters can be excitatory, in which case they increase neuronal activity, or they can be inhibitory, which "silences" neuronal activity. One of the most important excitatory neurotransmitters is glutamate, which can cause hyperexcitability in neurons in certain individuals, resulting in seizures. Seizures can also result from too little GABA in the brain, which is one of the most important inhibitory neurotransmitters (Henriques, 2016).

Indeed, epileptic seizures are the result of excessive electrical activity within the brain's neuronal networks. The research team conducted experimentation showing how acute fasting lowered synaptic activity at a neuromuscular junction, suggesting it may help prevent or reduce brain activity conducive to seizures in those predisposed. The team found that when food is unavailable, a protein called FOXO is activated, which promotes the expression of 4E-BP, a metabolic inhibitor. The research team believes that this research may demonstrate that fasting can dampen neuronal activity in a way that can reduce the severity of seizures (Henriques, 2016).

Indeed, fasting has been recommended as a treatment for seizures since the time of Hippocrates and also during the 1920s, and the ketogenic diet has sometimes been employed to alleviate symptoms in patients who do not have a lesion that can be resected surgically (Hartman et. al, 2014). In one attempt to replicate this alleged effect, researchers implemented an intermittent fasting regimen in six children, three of whom adhered to a combined regimen including both intermittent fasting and ketogenic diet for 2 months. Four of these children had transient improvement in seizure control, although they struggled with the hunger often associated with such an approach. The use of intermittent fasting protocols, perhaps in conjunction with the ketogenic diet, may be promising for seizure patients who do not respond to anticonvulsant medication, which is only effective for around two-thirds of patients.

Intriguingly, the ketogenic diet and intermittent fasting, although both apparently effective in reducing the severity of seizures, do not appear to share the same causal mechanisms in reducing this severity. (Hartman et. al, 2014). Ketogenic diet has shown to be helpful in reducing seizure activity, not only in humans, but also in mice, although intermittent fasting was found to lower the seizure threshold in mice. At this time, the exact mechanism by which intermittent fasting and the ketogenic protocols impact seizure activity remains unknown.

Perhaps surprisingly, some research suggests that intermittent fasting may reduce the symptoms of psoriasis. One study of 108 patients with moderate-to-severe plaque psoriasis who fasted during the month of Ramadan exhibited a significant decrease in Psoriasis Area and Severity Index (PASI) scores after this session of fasting. The same researchers also studied the effects of fasting on 37 individuals with psoriatic arthritis and found a similar decrease in the severity of symptoms. A 2018 review of nutritional strategies for psoriasis likewise found that weight loss and a healthy lifestyle notably reduced these same PASI scores among those with moderate-to-severe psoriasis, with low-calorie diets and intermittent fasting mitigating these symptoms among those who suffer from other conditions along with psoriasis (Morengo, 2020).

## Types of Intermittent Fasting

One of the more structured protocols for intermittent fasting is known as the 16/8 method, created as the "Leangains protocol" by fitness expert Martin Berkhan, which, as the name suggests, entails fasting every day for approximately 16 hours a day and restricting food consumption to the remaining 8 hours left in the day, give or take a couple hours. During this time, consumption of two or three meals is recommended (Gunnars, 2020). The simplest way of carrying out this method involves simply skipping breakfast and not eating anything after dinner. Dedicating the eating window to junk food consumption, however, will have the opposite of its intended effect, and so it is important to consume healthy food during this period (this, of course, is true of intermittent fasting methods for general, and is recommended when it comes to food consumption in general). Generally speaking, the method recommends 16 hours of fasting for men and 14-15 hours for women (Gunnars, 2020).

It is up to the individual as to how frequently they would like to repeat this cycle. Some choose to do it every single day, whereas others prefer to do it only once or twice a week. Indeed, it is this flexibility that makes it more popular than many other diet plans. Although a great deal of leeway is available to those who choose to participate in this dietary plan, it is generally recommended that the individual consume several small, healthy meals and snacks spaced evenly throughout the day in order to ensure that blood sugar remains stabilized and food cravings remain under control. The use of nutrient-rich foods is particularly important, and Health line recommends fruits such as apples, berries, oranges, bananas, pears and peaches, vegetables such as cauliflower, broccoli, cucumbers, tomatoes and leafy greens, whole grains such as rice, oats, barley, quinoa and black sweet, healthy fats such as avocados, coconut oil and olive oil, and sources of protein in the form of meat, fish, poultry, legumes, nuts, seeds and eggs. Calorie-free beverages such as water, unsweetened tea and coffee are helpful, and may allow you to curb your appetite while also remaining hydrated. As usual, it is important to avoid processed foods and junk food (Gunnars, 2020).

A great deal of research has demonstrated the health benefits of this form of fasting. Not only has this method of cutting calories been showing to boost metabolism and increase weight loss, but it has also been proven to reduce fasting insulin levels by up to 31 percent and lower blood sugar by 3-6 percent, suggesting that it may reduce one's risk for diabetes. Furthermore, animal studies suggest that it may increase life span (Gunnars, 2020).

Of course, restricting food intake to only 8 hours a day can tempt some people to eat more than usual during their food consumption periods, offsetting the benefits of fasting, which can lead to weight gain and digestive problems. Negative short-term effects in those susceptible may lead to weakness, hunger and fatigue. As noted before, this method of food restriction may impact males and females differently, and could interfere with the fertility of certain females (Gunnars, 2020). Apart from these caveats, the 16/8 intermittent fasting protocol is ordinarily a safe and easy way to improve health, provided the individual is consuming healthy foods during eating periods and living a healthy lifestyle in general. Nevertheless, it is important to speak with your physician if you are on any medications, have diabetes, a history of disordered eating, or struggle with low blood pressure. As usual, women who are trying to conceive, or those

9

who are pregnant or breastfeeding, should avoid such dietary restrictions.

Next is the "Warrior Diet," popularized by fitness expert Ori Hofmekler, which involves eating small amounts of raw fruits and vegetables during the day, followed by having a large meal at night. Although "fasting" is commonly understood in popular culture as total abstention from all eating, eating small amounts of raw fruit and vegetables throughout the day does technically count as a form of intermittent fasting. Those familiar with the paleo diet may already be familiar with protocols involving consumption of mostly whole, unprocessed food (Gunnars, 2020).

This diet derives its provocative name from being based on the alleged food consumption patterns of ancient warriors, who consumed little during the day and then feasted at night. Its founder argues that it functions by stressing the body deliberately through reduced food intake, which triggers its survival instincts. Nevertheless, the founder of the diet, Ori Hofmekler, emphasizes that this protocol is not based strictly on scientific experimentation but on his own observations (Gunnars, 2020). Those who follow this protocol are encouraged to consume small amounts of dairy products, raw fruit, hard-boiled eggs, vegetables and non-caloric fluids, during their 20-hour undereating session. After this, the dieter can binge on whatever they prefer during a four-hour feasting period. As usual, however, healthy and organic food choices are encouraged, and junk foods are discouraged. Those who follow this plan claim that it burns fat, increases energy levels, stimulates cellular repair and improves concentration.

Although there is no formally conducted scientific research to support this method, it is a form of intermittent fasting (which does have a great deal of scientific research backing its efficacy) and is more or less simply a more extreme version of the method. It would perhaps not be entirely inaccurate to refer to it as the 20:4 method. Indeed, other versions of 20-hour fasting cycles actually have been linked with weight loss. One protocol, although it did not correspond precisely with the so-called warrior diet, found that those who consumed meals over four hours in the evening actually experienced more weight loss than those who consumed the same number of calories throughout the day (Gunnars, 2020).

These individuals demonstrated significant reductions in fat mass, along with greater muscle mass. Other research on individuals with type 2 diabetes who engaged in a fasting protocol of between 18-20 hours a day found a major decrease in body weight and highly improved blood sugar control after fasting and after meals. The danger, of course, is that some who participate in this diet may end up consuming too many calories during the four-hour overeating period, thus offsetting any potential benefits of the fasting period (Gunnars, 2020). Indeed, this is an extreme form of intermittent fasting and it is quite difficult for many partakers to adhere to consistently. Individuals who should avoid this diet include children, women who are pregnant or nursing, those with type 1 diabetes, heart failure or certain cancers, individuals with disordered eating or who have a history of struggling with disordered eating, those who are already underweight, and extreme athletes.

Even those who do not struggle with disordered eating may develop unhealthy eating behaviors and have sometimes been observed resorting to binging and purging. Side effects of this extreme variant of intermittent fasting may include extreme hunger, insomnia, low energy, dizziness, fatigue, anxiety, constipation, hypoglycemia, weight gain, irritability and hormonal imbalances. Although those who plan appropriately during this fasting protocol and ensure that they consume a healthy amount of nutrient-dense foods, some health professionals likewise warn against this form of intermittent fasting on the grounds that they do not think those who participate in it will get enough nutrients.

Hofmekler recommends that those beginning with this diet ought to follow a three-week plan to ensure that the body is best able to transform its fat into energy. During Phase I / Week I, he recommends that the faster under eat for 20 hours during the day while consuming vegetable juices, dairy, clear broth, hard-boiled eggs and raw fruits and vegetables. During the four-hour feasting period, he recommends a salad with oil and vinegar dressing and then large amounts of plant proteins, small amounts of cheese and cooked vegetables, and wheat-free whole grains. Coffee, water, tea and small amounts of milk are allowed throughout the day during this period.

Phase II / Week II is similar to the first phase/week cycle, except instead of consuming plant protein during the four-hour feasting period, he recommends lean animal protein and at least one handful of nuts, accompanied by cooked vegetables. Grains and starches are to be avoided during this period. Finally, during Phase III / Week III, he recommends cycling between periods of high levels of carbohydrates and high levels of protein intake. This involves 1-2 days high in carbohydrates, 1-2 days high in protein and low in carbohydrates, 1-2 days high in carbohydrates once again, and 1-2 days high in protein and low in carbohydrates again. On the high-carbohydrate days, he recommends the standard 20-hour undereating protocol, followed by a four-hour feasting period with the aforementioned salad with oil and vinegar dressing, followed by cooked vegetables, then small amounts of animal protein, along with one main carbohydrate. This carb may come in the form of potatoes, pasta, corn, barley or oats.

On the other hand, during the high-protein / low-carbohydrate days, he recommends the standard 20-hour under eating protocol, followed by a four-hour feasting period involving a salad with oil and vinegar dressing, 8-16 ounces of animal protein accompanied with cooked, non-starchy vegetables, and then a small amount of fresh tropical fruit for dessert. During this stage, he recommends against grains or starches. After having completed these three phases, he recommends that the dieters should begin again. Hofmekler suggests that those undergoing this regimen take a daily multivitamin, other supplements and that they also do well to incorporate other healthy practices such as abundant water consumption and daily exercise.

Then there is the "Eat Stop Eat" protocol, articulated by fitness expert Brad Pilon, which involves total abstention from food intake for a full 24 hours following your last meal. After you have had breakfast, lunch or dinner, do not eat at all for the next 24 hours, and after this, you may resume food consumption as normal (Gunnars, 2020). Put simply, after you have finished dinner one night, do not eat at all until that time the next day. At this point, you will have completed a full, 24-hour fast and it is recommended, according to this protocol, to fast in such a way twice a week. Water, coffee and any other zero-calorie beverages are permitted during the fasting periods, but not solid food. Of course, it is important to eat the same amount of food during the food consumption periods as you would if you had not been fasting at all, and it is also important that this food intake is healthy.

Pilon markets this approach as a unique method of reevaluating "commonsense" understanding of meal timing and frequency in relation to your health, rather than as just another dietary fad. Although there is no direct scientific evidence for this specific protocol, the sort of prolonged fasting that the method employs is similar to other forms of intermittent fasting that have been scientifically proven as effective protocols. The main mechanism of action for this protocol is a deliberately induced caloric deficit that causes you to burn more calories than you consume. Nevertheless, evidence suggests that restricting calories for an entire day at a time, although certainly effective, is no more effective than other forms of more moderate, daily calorie restriction used by other protocols. Nevertheless, this method is designed to induce metabolic shifts that are conducive to weight loss and further research is required in order to understand how metabolic changes that may occur on this protocol can produce desired fat reduction.

Importantly, some individuals may have a hard time meeting daily nutrition needs on this diet, and it is therefore particularly important for those who choose this protocol to pay close attention to the foods they consume on non-fasting days, in order to ensure that they consume enough protein, vitamins, minerals and fiber throughout their diet. Those who require unusually high amounts of nutrition may want to consider other more moderate protocols in order to ensure that they avoid unhealthy weight loss. Those with diabetes in particular may experience dangerously low levels of blood sugar on this protocol, and may want to consider alternative methods of healthy food consumption (Gunnars, 2020). This is also true of those who take prescription blood sugar medications or who have medical conditions that cause poor blood sugar regulation. Even ordinarily healthy people may experience unwanted side effects such as irritability, mood instability and reduced libido. This protocol is furthermore contraindicated among those with a history of disordered eating or those with a tendency towards developing unhealthy or disordered eating patterns.

The "Eat Stop Eat" diet is one variant of what is known as alternate day fasting. According to this protocol, you eat whatever you want on non-fasting days but abstain to varying degrees on fasting days. Although the variant of this which we have just examined is one of the more extreme variants, one form of this method of intermittent fasting allows you to eat 500 calories on fasting days. Fasting days, as is usually the case, allows water, unsweetened coffee and tea, and those who are using the modified version which allows 500 calories on fasting days receive 20-25 percent of their energy requirements.

Although Pilon's variant is quite popular, the most popular form of this method of intermittent fasting is Dr. Krista Varady's "Every Other Day Diet." In addition to having pioneered this most popular method of alternate day fasting, she has also conducted the most research on it. Dr. Varady's protocol, which is less extreme than Pilon's, allows consumption of a small percentage of one's daily energy requirements (about 500 calories) on fasting days, and these fasting-day nutrients can be consumed whether at lunch or dinner, yielding the same benefits either way.

One of the most widely celebrated benefits of this form of fasting, is that it is far easier to stick to than everyday caloric restriction. This may be the result of the protocol generating optimal amounts of the satiety hormone leptin and the hunger hormone ghrelin as a result of this pattern (Bjarnadottir, 2020). Indeed, research on animals suggests that modified forms of alternate day fasting resulted in decreased levels of these hunger hormones and increased levels of satiety hormones compared to other forms of intermittent fasting. Although there is some inconsistency when it comes to the impact of this diet on "compensatory hunger" (increased levels of hunger as a result of calorie restriction), much of the research suggests that alternate day fasting does not increase compensatory hunger as much as continuous calorie restriction, and even individuals who do tend to struggle initially with compensatory hunger often claim that their hunger levels diminish after approximately the first two weeks, eventually resulting in almost effortless fasting activity (Bjarnadottir, 2020). Although ADF and daily calorie restriction have both been shown to be equally effective at reducing harmful belly fat and inflammation markers in obese individuals, therefore, this form of intermittent fasting has the

15

added psychological appeal of being easier to adhere to than other protocols. Nevertheless, other research suggests that alternate day fasting may be better than daily calorie restriction diets because it generates greater fat loss and preserves muscle mass.

One of the reasons for the superior tolerability of the alternate day fasting approach relative to other forms of intermittent fasting is its tendency to not cause a certain kind of drop in metabolic rate that is characteristic of other forms of intermittent fasting. Severely restricting one's caloric intake through continuous caloric restriction causes the body to begin to conserve energy by reducing the number of calories it burns (Bjarnadottir, 2020). Alternate day fasting, however, does not have this effect and only reduces resting metabolic rate by 1 percent, as opposed to methods of continuous calorie restriction, which decreases resting metabolic rate by 6 percent. Indeed, even after 24 unsupervised weeks of continuous calorie restriction, this group still had a resting metabolic rate of 4.5 percent, while those who had participated in the alternate-day fasting had resting metabolic rates that were normal.

In general, research on overweight and obese adults shows that it is possible to lose up to 3-8 percent of your body weight in only 2-12 weeks with this form of intermittent fasting, and it is especially effective among middle-aged individuals. This is especially true, according to recent research, when this method is combined with endurance exercise, as this may lead to twice as much weight loss than practicing alternate day fasting alone and may even generate as much as six times as much weight loss as endurance exercise in isolation. In fact, alternate day fasting appears to be equally effective whether you are eating a low-fat or a high-fat diet (Bjarnadottir, 2020).

Alternate day fasting does more, however, than simply eliminating unwanted fat. Instead, it appears to actually have qualitatively unique effects on your body composition compared with other forms of

16

fasting. Although research suggests that traditional methods of calorie restriction and alternate day fasting are equally effective at getting rid of weight and fat mass, alternate day fasting is unique in its ability to preserve muscle mass; a form of weight that you do not want to lose (Bjarnadottir, 2020). Indeed, if you are losing both muscle mass and fat then you are decreasing the number of calories burnt by your body daily, which defeats the whole purpose of weight loss regimens. In one study comparing alternate day fasting with another more conventional form of calorie restriction, the researchers observed that the ADF group had preserved a great deal more muscle and had also lost more fat than the other group (Bjarnadottir, 2020).

Research suggests that alternate day fasting is the most effective means of intermittent fasting when it comes to reducing insulin levels and insulin resistance, suggesting a protective effect against type 2 diabetes as well as other chronic diseases such as heart disease and cancer. Furthermore, individuals with prediabetes who undergo 8-12 weeks of alternate day fasting have demonstrated a decrease in fasting insulin levels by an astonishing 20-31 percent. This protocol has also shown to decrease blood pressure, reduce bad cholesterol and triglycerides and reduce waist circumference (Bjarnadottir, 2020). Health benefits are evident in animal studies as well, demonstrating delayed aging, reduced risk of tumors, and both long-term and short-term inducement of autophagy, which is attended with numerous health benefits.

Alternate-day fasting is beneficial for weight loss in both obese and non-obese individuals. One study that followed non-obese individuals on this regimen for 3-weeks found that the diet decreased fasting insulin, increased fat burning, and led to a 4 percent decrease in fat mass. Since hunger remained quite high during this study, the researchers suggested that the modified alternate-day fasting mentioned above, which allows one small meal on fasting days, might

17

improve tolerability for those who do not struggle with obesity (Bjarnadottir, 2020). Another study that compared the impact of this diet on overweight individuals and those within a more normal weight range found that following the alternate day fasting regimen for 12 weeks led to a decrease in fat mass and also improved variables related to risk of heart disease. It is important to understand, however, that this diet is specifically for those looking to lose weight or fat mass, and so those with other goals in mind might want to try another regimen (Bjarnadottir, 2020).

Whether you are following the modified form of the alternate day fasting approach that allows 500 calories a day, or the more extreme version that requires a total 24 hour fast, it is permissible to drink non-calorie beverages such as unsweetened coffee, tea and water. Those allowing themselves 500 calories a day may prefer one large meal late in the day while others eat 2-3 small meals that add up to 500 calories. When you do eat, make sure to consume a great deal of high-protein and nutrient-dense foods, such as low-calorie vegetables, which will make you feel fuller without adding too many calories. Other recommended foods for fasting days include grilled fish or lean meat with vegetables, yogurt with berries, soup and fruit or a combination of eggs and vegetables. As usual, children, pregnant and lactating women, those with certain medical conditions and those with eating disorders or struggling with unusually low body weight, should not partake in this or any other fasting regimen. Those uncertain as to whether they fall into any of these categories ought to consult with a physician especially if they are currently taking any medications.

One form of intermittent fasting, known as the 5:2 diet, recommends eating normally for 5 days of the week while restricting caloric intake to 500-600 calories for the remaining two (500 for women and 600 for men). Popularized by British journalist Michael Mosley, it is also known as the Fast Diet and suggests that for your two fasting days, you consume 2 small meals of 250 calories (in the case of women) or 300 calories (in the case of men) (Gunnars, 2020). Although this particular form of intermittent fasting remains relatively understudied compared with other popular forms, animal studies have certainly been suggestive in its favor. Research has found through animal studies that this form of intermittent fasting produced a reduction in fat tissue, as well as cells that store this fat, and has also found that this protocol is just as effective as ordinary calorie restriction with respect to improvement of metabolic health and weight loss.

Those who partake in this diet are encouraged to cut caloric intake to 25 percent of their otherwise ordinary intake on the relevant fast days. For example, someone who eats about 2,000 calories a day should eat around 500 calories on their fast days. Many people prefer to space out their fasting days rather than making them consecutive, which makes the protocol much easier to adhere to due to lower psychological strain of continually low caloric intake. Those who conduct the diet in this way oftentimes feel more satisfied with their diet since they do not feel chronically deprived of the foods they enjoy and the energy these foods confer (Gunnars, 2020). Due to this more moderate approach to fasting and dieting, many of those who participate in it find that it is a simple and straightforward method of restricting calories and thus burning fat.

This form of fasting allows for a great deal of flexibility and apart from the broad, general recommendations that distinguishes it from other dietary plans, allows the individual to conduct himself in a way he feels most comfortable. As long as you are consuming only 25 percent of your ordinary caloric intake on the relevant days, and you are consistently eating in a healthy manner, you should expect the diet to have its intended effects. Some people may elect to start the day with a small breakfast to energize their body for the day, whereas others may feel it is more appropriate or comfortable for them to skip breakfast altogether on the grounds that eating breakfast may cause them to feel hungrier throughout the day and make the diet more difficult. For such people, it may be more appropriate to begin food consumption with a healthy lunch rather than breakfast. You might eat three small meals during the day, or an early lunch and dinner, a single meal at dinner or breakfast, or eat a small breakfast and late lunch while foregoing dinner. Any of these strategies, as long as conducted in moderation, with healthy food and in accordance with the caloric recommendation, ought to have the intended effects of the diet.

That said, it is important to keep the body satisfied on fast days. Since you are consuming only small amounts of food on these days, it is recommended that you consume foods that have a great deal of nutrients, including fiber and protein. Eating vegetables on fast days may help the individual feel more well-fed in spite of the relatively meager caloric intake, since it is possible to consume a great deal of vegetables within a small meal without consuming very many calories at all. Vegetables consisting of dark, leafy greens and salads are especially recommended, and may add to the sense of feeling full without actually being too full of calories. Medical News Today recommends using a spiralizer to turn zucchini or carrots into noodles, producing a healthy and tasty sauce that can accompany the smaller fasting meals. They also recommend ensuring that plenty of protein is consumed, and without too much fat, which can be accomplished with eggs, lean animal cuts, white fish, tofu, beans, peas and lentils.

They also recommend dark berries, such as blueberries and blackberries, in order to provide the kind of natural sugar that will allay the kinds of sweet cravings that can lead the tempted faster to compromise restrictions on caloric intake. Other recommendations include soup, since the added water and broth spices make the individual feel fuller without the added calories, plenty of water in order to stave off the hunger pains, and plain and unsweetened coffee and tea. During fast days, it is important to avoid processed foods, which usually contain a large number of calories, the excess fats that come with cooking oils, cheese and animal fats, and carbohydrates found in breads, white rice and pastas. As an example of the sort of meal recommended for fast days, they suggest vegetable soup with a side of hard-boiled eggs, a small cut of steamed white fish, a large portion of steamed vegetables with spices and salts, combined with another large portion of salad with fresh vegetables (Gunnars, 2020).

## Fasting and Your Body

In order to fully appreciate the benefits of fasting, it is important to understand the biological basis of these benefits. In fact, in scientific studies of fasting and caloric restriction that is modest enough to avoid malnutrition have consistently been found to produce a variety of health effects, not only in humans, but across many species, including non-human primates. For example, in one study, mice who were subjected to time-restricted feeding involving 40% caloric restriction were protected from decline in muscle mass normally associated with aging (Anton et al., 2018). This is quite contrary to the stereotype of those who engage in fasting as emaciated and lacking in healthy musculature! Furthermore, when these mice were fed high-fat diets, they only become obese if they do not undergo alternate diet fasting, whereas if they were subjected to this protocol, they avoided obesity and also retained their muscle mass (Anton et al., 2018).

This protocol of time restricted feeding entailed an eating pattern in which food intake was restricted to specific time periods of the day, usually between 8-12 hours a day. Remarkably, rats subjected to alternate day fasting protocols, which involve eating patterns in which no calories are consumed on fasting days, after which the rats are treated to a "feast" day without food intake restriction, experienced an average lifespan increased by 30 percent. These rats consistently maintained a lower body weight and were able to enjoy a higher level of daily running when provided with running wheels, compared with rats who did not undergo any caloric restriction.

These health benefits are quite evident in overweight humans, in whom short-term caloric restriction (for around six months) can significantly improve multiple health risk factors. The health benefits observed include an astonishing array of biological effects, including improvements in osteoarthritis, healing of otherwise refractory dermal ulcers and thrombophlebitis, mitochondrial function, dyslipidemia, inflammation cytokines, insulin-sensitivity and, of course, cardiovascular risk factors, as well as improving tolerance of elective surgery (Anton et al., 2018).

Understanding the biological basis of improvements in these biological pathways requires understanding the nature of the "metabolic switch" that is flipped when the individual undergoes intermittent fasting; a switch that occurs between 12 to 36 hours after the individual ceases' food consumption. This switch refers to the decision of both the body and the brain to use fatty acids and fatty acid-derived ketones for fuel rather than glucose; a switch that is observed during periods of extended exercise and also during fasting (Anton et al., 2018).

When this switch is flipped, the body begins to resort to fat in the form of free fatty acids (FFAs) and fatty-acid derived ketones rather than through the synthesis of lipids. Ketones are simply chemicals produced by your liver which are generated when your body does not have enough insulin to turn sugar into energy. Your body resorts to fat instead, and the liver turns this fat into ketones, a form of acid, that is then released into your bloodstream, allowing muscles and other tissues to use them for fuel (Anton et al., 2018).

Once this switch is flipped, there is a shift from fat storage to mobilization of fat in the form of free fatty acids (FFAs) and fatty-acid derived ketones. The glycogen of the liver cells no longer provides the energy they once did during this period, and fat tissue is burned up at an accelerated rate. Ordinarily, glycogen is deposited in liver cells and functions as an energy reserve that can be quickly mobilized to meet sudden needs (Anton et al., 2018). Within liver cells, this substance can make up around 8% of liver weight, and it is the depletion of these reserves that functions as an inflection point which triggers the metabolic shift sought after in intermittent fasting. Exactly how long it takes for this metabolic switch to occur depends on the glycogen content of the liver at the time of the onset of the fast, as well as how much energy the individual is using (Anton et al., 2018). For this reason, exercise may expedite the process of the metabolic switch, and the individual who may want to quicken and enhance the effects of fasting may want to supplement the practice with exercise.

FFAs are eventually transported to liver cells where they are metabolized by β-oxidation to produce the ketones that eventually become available as energy sources. These ketones are then sent en masse to cells that require high levels of energy due to their high metabolic activity, such as muscle cells and neurons where they are turned into acetyl coenzyme A (Anton et al., 2018). This substance is then used to produce adenosine triphosphate, which is an organic compound that provides energy which guides many processes found in all sorts of living cells and is very important when it comes to intracellular energy transfer (Anton et al., 2018).

Research suggests that it is precisely this shift from fatty acid to ketone oxidation (instead of glucose oxidation) that may be responsible for preservation of muscle mass. Muscle cells contain triglycerides in little lipid droplets, which provide a readily accessible source of fatty acids. These fatty acids are used for ketone generation, the preferred energy source of the brain and body; a process useful for both extended periods of fasting as well as exercise (Anton et al., 2018). A transcriptional regulator called PPAR-α activates expression of genes that assist in the oxidation of fatty acids in muscle cells. It is these genes that assist in the shift in muscle cell preference for fatty acids, instead of their reliance on glucose, during both fasting and intense exercise. Research in mice with these genes inactivated exhibit lower levels of oxidative fibers in certain of their muscles, whereas overexpression of this gene increases the number of such fibers. Remarkably, mice who have been biologically modified in a similar way are intolerant of exercise and their muscle cells do not adapt to exercise the way healthy, typical mice do (Anton et al., 2018).

For these and related reasons, experts have begun to suggest intermittent fasting regimens may be helpful in treating both obesity and other related metabolic conditions, including metabolic syndrome and even type 2 diabetes. Indeed, since intermittent fasting has been found to improve conditions related to insulin sensitivity, it should come as no surprise that it helps type 2 diabetes, which is characterized precisely by a lack thereof. Unfortunately, these benefits may be notoriously absent from your typical Westerner, whose diet ordinarily prohibits the flip of this metabolic switch that would ordinarily produce these health benefits.

In fact, studies conducted as early as 1914 have used fasting as an allegedly effective treatment for both type 1 and type 2 diabetes, with many subsequent studies replicating these results. One study even reported a severely obese woman who experienced resolution of her diabetes following only one month of fasting, leading to normal glucose tolerance for over a year after she regained the weight. Several other studies have found enhanced insulin sensitivity and glucose tolerance for those with diabetes almost immediately following a fast. Nevertheless, of course, fasting with diabetes can be risky and anyone with either form of diabetes who is interested in pursuing a fasting regimen of any sort ought to consult with his or her physician before attempting this.

## Fasting and Your Mind

We are all familiar with the complaint of the individual who has gone too long without eating and whose head is therefore foggy from lack of nutrition. Nevertheless, it may come as a surprise to readers that a great deal of research has emerged suggesting that specific fasting protocols may contribute to greater brain health and may actually prevent cognitive decline, rather than cause it. In fact, studies of mice on time restricted feeding and caloric intake regimens suggest that these protocols significantly reduced the severity of otherwise predictable declines in motor performance and maze learning as the mice began to reach an advanced age (Anton et al., 2018). Although it is not clear at this time what accounts for the biological basis of this preservation of brain health through fasting, it is possible that the preference of the brain for ketone utilization may be one of the operative mechanisms, as it may prevent age-related reductions in white matter.

Other research has suggested that similar methods of caloric restrictions enhance or preserve the health of the hippocampus in mice; a brain region we share with them which is very important for learning and memory. Increase in synapse numbers in this part of the brain is likewise correlated with increased levels of brain-derived neurotrophic factor (BDNF), which is one of the substances in the brain responsible for the efficacy of antidepressants and exercise in reducing depression and anxiety. This is one respect in which many ancient religious and spiritual interpretations of the significance of fasting may have long anticipated the therapeutic impact of fasting on the human mind, even if they were not yet able to examine the biological pathways and causal mechanisms which mediate these effects (Anton et al., 2018).

In fact, independent research on the impact of caloric restriction specifically on major depressive disorder suggests that at least some of these regimens may improve depressive symptoms. Despite having helped a great many people, antidepressants do not work for everyone, and intermittent fasting, which mediates antidepressant effects in a manner that overlaps with that of the medication often used for this disorder, has shown some degree of clinical efficacy in treating these symptoms. It is unclear, however, exactly how these effects are mediated in caloric restriction, although some research suggests that ketone production may be involved. Indeed, it is possible that multiple biological pathways are involved in ways that are poorly understood at this time and many-layered.

Other research suggests that "ghrelin," the so-called hunger hormone, may be instrumental in producing the antidepressant effects of intermittent fasting. One study in the journal Molecular Psychiatry found that ghrelin is a natural antidepressant that promotes neurogenesis. Predictably, ghrelin levels increase in times of fasting, and this correlation suggests that this hormone may function as one of the causal mechanisms involved in improving depression symptoms through intermittent fasting.

As in the aforementioned animal models, research conducted on the impact of fasting on the brain in humans suggests that the positive effects appear regardless of age. One study, for example, reported that fasting and caloric restriction profoundly relieved negative emotional states such as anger, tension and confusion in aging men, and even generated a sense of euphoria; an effect which some researchers believe may be linked to endorphin secretion resulting from fasting; an effect that is particularly notable in the practitioner during the first 48 hours of onset (Zhang et. al, 2015). Caloric restriction has even been shown in some research to mitigate the severity of the effects of chronic pain after undergoing a protocol of 250kcal/day for 2 weeks, leading to an improvement in depressive mood among 80 percent of the patients (Zhang et. al, 2015).

Similar effects of calorie restriction on depressive symptoms were observed in animal studies. Mice subjected to calorie restriction became more socially active than control mice in one experiment, and it is possible that the tendency of calorie restriction to protect against neuron degeneration may be at least partially responsible for this effect (Zhang et. al, 2015). Indeed, some research has suggested that depression may actually be better understood as a subtle neurodegenerative disorder rather than most fundamentally as a mood disorder. Postmortem and imaging studies consistently neuronal atrophy and death in the prefrontal cortices and hippocampi of clinically depressed patients. This provides an interesting parallel between the neurological and behavioral consequences of depression for the hippocampus in both humans and mice, and likewise, an interesting parallel in the mechanism by which such negative consequences might be prevented. Other studies suggest that antidepressants may protect against this atrophy, and since fasting appears to be capable of a similar impact, it may be that future research will lead scientists to conclude suggesting fasting as a supplemental treatment to depression alongside medication.

In these respects, evidence begins to emerge that fasting enhances both cognitive and emotional centers of the brain, increases health in both domains and may likewise protect against negative consequences, or even repair the damage resulting from them. Other research likewise shows that although many cognitive traits and characteristics are highly heritable, gene expression responsible for this variation can be either inhibited or promoted depending on certain environmental factors. Research on caloric restriction and time-restricted feeding may enhance the expressivity of these genes and thus enhance the capacity of the brain's neuroplasticity in certain cognitive domains. In other words, suppose a gene variant is discovered that appears to be positively correlated with better memory in mice or humans. The beneficial impact of this variant might only show up if the body to which it belongs takes adequate care of itself or is properly nurtured in a healthy environment. The complex interaction between genes and environment has emerged as a topic of great interest among scientists in both the social and the physical sciences, and food consumption appears to play an important role in this domain.

Alternate day fasting in particular has also shown to improve cognitive function in mice (Zhang et. al, 2015). In one study, when mice were subjected to such a diet for 6-8 months, their performance on memory and learning tasks was significantly enhanced compared to control mice who were fed every day instead of alternating daily between fasting and feeding. Another study subjected 20-month-old mice to such a diet for 3 months and likewise found that their learning and memory performance on a water maze test was significantly enhanced. These experiments combined show that these effects are measurable whether the mice are subjected to the regimen early on in their formative years, as well as later in life.

This dietary pattern has been shown in similar animal models to protect neurons from dysfunction in mice with a wide range of neurological diseases and disorders and other forms of brain injury, such as stroke, Alzheimer's disease, epilepsy and Parkinson's disease. Mice who were placed on such a regimen, in one study, were subjected to a focal ischemic stroke, but those mice who were subjected to this dietary model had the impact of their brain damage significantly mitigated compared to those who were fed daily. The researchers were led to believe that the ketone β-OHB was involved in mediating this effect, since it is well-known that it can suppress epileptic seizures and emerging research suggests it may exhibit neuroprotective effects in other diseases as well, such as Alzheimer's disease, stroke and Parkinson's disease.

# Around the World

Few spiritual practices are as universally prevalent among ancient world religions as the practice of fasting. In this section, we will take a brief look at the rich diversity present among some of the more prominent spiritual traditions of the world in which fasting is regarded as an important part of how they understand and practice contact with the divine.

## Hinduism

Strictly speaking, the terms "Hindu" and "Hinduism" were coined by ancient Persians and Greeks who coined them after initially encountering indigenous people following this religion along the river Indus in India. After this, 19th century British academics added the suffix "-ism" to the words as they gained acceptance in everyday language. However, the belief system is properly classified by its practitioners as Sanātana Dharma, meaning "eternal law" or "eternal way." Hindus refer to their conception of the ultimate divine being or state of being as "Brahman," which can also be translated "God" or "Absolute." There is a great deal of diversity, however, among Hindus, concerning how the divine should be understood, with some Hindus conceiving of the Divine as pervading the entire universe to the point of being ultimately inseparable from it (a form of either pantheism or panentheism), whereas others conceive of Brahman as something more transcendent and having a component that is outside of space and time.

The Vedas are the authoritative body of scripture for Hindus and provide the instructions and rationale for fasting. These accounts emphasize both the physical and spiritual benefits of fasting, as the practice is seen as a cleansing ritual for both body and spirit, and Hindus believe this helps the practitioner become closer to God and also to counter potentially negative forces. Fasting is also used for purely ritual purposes, both as a means of participation in life cycle sacraments and as a means of participating in holy days and festivals, such as Navarātrī, a nine-night celebration that occurs five times a year ("Hindu Fasting in the Workplace," 2019).

Due to the great diversity of Hindu beliefs, there is great variation when it comes to when Hindus choose to fast. When they choose to do so depends to a great degree upon which god they choose to worship in their formidable pantheon. For example, devotees of Lord Śiva often fast on Mondays, while devotees of Lord Vishnu are more likely to fast on Thursdays. Fasting is also sometimes used by Hindus as a means of repentance, whose purpose is to cleanse the individual of past sins, and also to enhance impulse control and master the passions, in order to prevent the individual from becoming guilty of further sin. Some forms of fasting in Hinduism may seem quite extreme by modern Western standards, and can involve intense restriction on consumption of both food and water for a certain number of days, whereas other forms are more moderate and may involve eating and drinking (or abstaining from) only certain types of food and drink for a certain number of days.

## Buddhism

Fasting in Buddhism has some solemn beginnings. It is believed by Buddhists that the Buddha attempted to live on only one grain of rice a day for an extended period of time, prior to giving up this excessively austere lifestyle for more moderate practices; a realization that preceded his moment of awakening or Enlightenment. He realized that such an extreme practice would cause him to die prior to reaching Enlightenment and that it was therefore counterproductive, aside from depriving him of the strength to properly meditate. It was after he was provided nourishment by a sympathetic woman that he regained his strength and decided to practice what came to be known as "The Middle Way"; an intermediate between the extremes of severe austerity and unrestricted indulgence.

One of the oldest traditions of Buddhism, Theravada Buddhism, takes its doctrine concerning fasting from the so-called "Tipitaka," a Pali term meaning "three baskets", so-called because of its tripartite division. It is in these texts that we find codified the teaching that it is impossible to achieve wisdom through forms of fasting that are taken to an unhealthy extreme. Fasting should be done healthily and in moderation, and not as a form of self-punishment. Monks in this tradition eat a light breakfast and then abstain from food until noon. Conducted in moderation, meditation functions as a means of improving the impact of meditation and can be found in all extant Buddhist schools, including Mahayana and Vajrayana traditions, whose monks consume two light vegetable meals a day during periods of fasting.

Among Buddhist monks, fasting is listed as a "dhutanga" practice, which means "to shake up" or to promote vigor (Gaikwad, 2017). There are 13 of such practices, 4 of which are related to food consumption. These recommendations state that the monk ought to eat once a day, reduce consumption, eat while sitting and only consume food that they receive at the initial seven households they consult. Nevertheless, fasting, in Buddhism, is not something that is coercively imposed on the individual but is conducted voluntarily.

31

Theravada Buddhists engage in an intriguing religious practice known as "vassa," whose purpose is to fast in order to deliberately produce and experience craving as a means of confronting the experiences of attachment and aversion, and using mindfulness to remain at ease even while the body remains in a state of want or discomfort (Gaikwad, 2017). This practice dovetails well with the overall goal of Theravada Buddhism as a means of extinguishing craving and attachment by remaining mindful of the experience of these undesirable emotional states without being controlled or dominated by them. By cultivating such an attitude towards life, Buddhists hope to one day be released from the wheel of reincarnation, characterized as it is by continual suffering.

Apart from the earlier Theravada tradition, later traditions expand upon and develop methods of fasting which are distinct from, but overlap with, the underlying principles embodied in early Buddhist theory and practice. For example, Mahayana Buddhists use fasting to purify both body and mind and to confront the experience of craving. As in the Theravada tradition, fasting is not a mandatory practice, but it is often practiced by monks. The fasting Mahayana Buddhist consumes only dry bread for 3 days in order to prepare themselves for a period of more extreme abstention from food in later fast days. These periods of fasting can be quite rigorous, ranging from 18 days to up to 72 days (Gaikwad, 2017).

Adherents of the Tibetan Vajrayana tradition engage in fasting periods of 2 days as part of the Nyungne ceremony, which involves chanting and meditation, with the aim of purifying the human body and reducing negative karma. During this ceremony, the first day involves consuming one vegetarian meal before noon that avoids garlic, radish, onions, eggs or any meat, although light liquids are permitted, provided no juices are consumed containing pulp. During the second day, nothing whatsoever can be consumed, whether food or drink, solid or liquid. Advocates of this tantric tradition use these methods to enhance certain special abilities of the human body, such as the ability to control body heat. As with the other traditions, fasting is not mandatory here (Gaikwad, 2017).

## Islam

Ramadan, the ninth month of the Islamic calendar, is observed by Muslims worldwide as a month of prayer, fasting and spiritual devotion. During this period, Muslims engage in dawn-to-dusk fasting combined with nightly feasts as a means of becoming closer to God and cultivating self-control. During this time, the Muslim believer is encouraged to detach himself from physical and temporal pleasure and devote oneself to prayer and spiritual disciplines. A rigorous period of fasting, abstention from eating and drinking from dawn to dusk endures for the entire month of Ramadan, and even the slightest sip of water is seen as a way of breaking the fast.

But Ramadan is about more than just fasting. It is a full-orbed method of cultivating deep and profound impulse control by abstaining from sexual intercourse during the day, avoidance of uncontrolled anger, fighting and uncontrolled emotional and volitional outbursts in general. During this period, Muslims are encouraged to observe the five daily prayers and to recite the Qur'an just before their fast ends each day at sunset. Preparation for the fast occurs during "suhoor," which is a pre-dawn meal whose purpose is to help them get through the day. Some are exempted from fasting, such as those who are sick, pregnant and menstruating women, children and the elderly.

## Christianity

Attitudes towards fasting vary widely within Christianity depending on sect or denomination of the individual devotee. Fasting tends to play a large role in Christianity in the more liturgical denominations of

Christianity, such as Roman Catholicism and Eastern Orthodoxy than it does in Western Protestantism. Perhaps surprisingly, the New Testament has very little to say explicitly about fasting. Although Jesus does give very brief instructions on how not to fast, when contrasting the inappropriate and ostentatious displays of the religious leaders of his day, who made a large show of their fasting to impress onlookers, Jesus does not actually command his disciples to fast, and it does not seem to have played a major role in his teaching. He does, however, assume his disciples would fast after his departure (Lk. 5:35). As an interesting exception to the otherwise apparent laxity when it comes to fasting in the New Testament, there is Jesus' fast of 40 days and 40 nights when he is described as having been tempted by Satan.

For Roman Catholics, Ash Wednesday and Good Friday are the only obligatory days of fasting. These norms of fasting are mandatory from age 18 until age 59. During this fast, the individual is permitted to eat a single full meal as well as two smaller meals, provided that together they do not equal a full meal. Abstinence from meat is binding on members of the Roman Catholic Church from age 14 onwards. The fast on Good Friday is continued until Easter Vigil (Holy Saturday Night). This is known as the "paschal fast" and its purpose is to honor the suffering and death of Jesus of Nazareth.

## Judaism

Although there are 25 holidays and events throughout the Jewish year associated with fasting, the practice is only mandatory on Yom Kippur, during which Jewish believers atone for their sins. Females over the age of 12 and males over the age of 13 are required to abstain from all food or drink for the duration of the holiday. Children under the age of 9 are not permitted to fast. Extenuating circumstances having to do with health are acknowledged in Judaism, and there is one well-known anecdote about a Rabbi commanding his whole congregation to eat on Yom Kippur during a cholera outbreak in order

34

to protect them from succumbing to the disease. Pregnant and nursing women are also discouraged from fasting.

## Jainism

Fasting is more important to Jain spirituality than it is to almost any other religious or spiritual tradition. Although practitioners of the ancient Indian religion Jainism may impose fasts upon themselves at any time, most Jains fast during special festivals or holy days during the year. Some Jain fasts are conducted for the purpose of penance. This is particularly true of monks and nuns. Fasting is seen as a means of purifying both the body and mind and recalls the tradition's emphasis on asceticism; a form of rigorous spirituality in which the individual is expected to renounce worldly comforts in favor of a life devoted exclusively to spiritual cultivation.

Jains take fasting very seriously, and have a specific purpose in mind when it is conducted. Instead of merely temporarily renouncing food consumption, the Jain is taught that he must stop wanting to eat altogether in order to mortify attachments to the temporal and physical world. If this underlying spiritual injunction is ignored, the practitioner of Jain spirituality sees fasting as pointless. Some give up both food and water completely for a certain period, and others simply eat less than is necessary to avoid hunger. Other forms of fasting within Jain spirituality include Vruti Sankshepa, which involves limiting the number of items consumed, and Rasa Parityaga, which involves giving up only favorite foods.

Some Jains engage in particularly extreme forms of fasting that might not be feasible for the average faster. Some, for example, fast for months at a time. Famously, Hira Ratan Manek is said to have fasted for over 6 months, whereas Sri Sahaj Muni Maharaj is said to have fasted for over a year, completing a record-breaking 365-day fast on May 1, 1998.

A particularly solemn form of fasting with which I am unfamiliar apart from Jainism is Santhara or Sallenkhana, which is a procedure in which a Jain stops eating with the intention of preparing to die. This is only done, however, when the body is in such a state of medical disrepair that the individual regards it as no longer functioning acceptably as a vehicle of spirituality and when death is an indisputable certainty, as in the case of a terminal illness. This is done with the intention to purify the body and remove attachments to the physical world from the mind. Those who undertake this practice are regarded as spiritual heroes by fellow Jains and their deaths are regarded as occasions of public celebrations, because when it is undertaken, it is seen as a means of eradicating all sin and bad karma and leading to ultimate cessation of the painful process of reincarnation into a new suffering body after death.

## Who Should Not Fast?

Even on non-fasting days, it is important to avoid or at least restrict many of the foods you would normally avoid on fast days. Individuals with low blood sugar or who easily feel fatigued or dizzy without eating might want to avoid this diet. Pregnant or breastfeeding women should avoid fasting, and children and teenagers ought to likewise avoid it apart from guidance from a physician, as their bodies are still in the process of developing. Likewise, those with chronic conditions, especially diabetes, should consult with a physician before attempting to engage in any fasting.

Fasting is not for everyone and may pose risks to certain particularly vulnerable groups, which include those suffering from certain physical and mental conditions. Those who are at risk for an eating disorder, or who actually suffer from an eating disorder, should not attempt to engage in fasting. Others who may be put at risk when fasting and engaging in related practices include, but may not be limited to, people with certain forms of chronic diseases, and individuals struggling with hypoglycemia.

And, of course, even for those of us who are not part of a high-risk group, fasting does pose certain difficulties such as low energy, irritability, temperature sensitivity, persistent hunger, and difficulty engaging in higher quality work and activity performance. Therefore, although it is certainly not impossible for someone working in construction to fast, such an individual may want to choose a protocol that entails food restriction intake on his days off rather than when he is involved in strenuous physical exertion as part of his daily occupation. Likewise, those engaged in occupations that involve high levels of complex mental computation may want to only engage in caloric restriction on their days off, to ensure the possibility of cognitive fatigue does not interfere with their work. Individuals engaged in an occupation characterized by high degrees of emotional strain may likewise want to either avoid intermittent fasting, or at least restrict fasting days to days off.

Although intermittent fasting has proven largely safe and beneficial in human and animal models, there are some dangers associated with the practice, and those who are psychologically or biologically predisposed to these potential risk factors should be particularly keen to consult with a physician before beginning. To those predisposed to certain tendencies, intermittent fasting may contribute to orthorexia, which should be understood as an obsession with proper eating. This may lead to a preoccupation with talking about your diet constantly and an unhealthy obsession with determining what to eat next. In this respect, intermittent fasting, for certain individuals, may find that their dietary pattern interferes with their social life. For example, some individuals may feel pressured to cancel social events on the grounds that the culinary options available are inconsistent with their dietary needs.

Of course, this is more of a subjective preference and it is on the individual to decide if he or she feels that these dietary habits are interfering with his or her life in a socially unhealthy way. Further psychological consequences may entail increased guilt, since those who may accidentally break their fast, or start it either too early or too late, may be susceptible to higher levels of guilt, anxiety or shame. Those who practice intermittent fasting should be aware that more extreme reactions of this sort may be signs of disordered eating patterns.

It is important to understand that intermittent fasting may sometimes be associated with significantly increased LDL levels. In one study, metabolically healthy obese adults who conducted alternate day fasting had much higher LDL levels than those who engaged in ordinary, daily calorie restriction. LDL is widely known as "bad" cholesterol, the waxy substance found in your blood. Although cholesterol is required in order to build healthy cells, abnormally high levels of this form of cholesterol can significantly increase one's risk of heart disease. These higher levels can eventually lead to fatty deposits in your blood levels, making it harder for enough blood to flow through these arteries. These deposits can sometimes break suddenly, forming a clot that can lead to either a heart attack or a stroke. LDL, which stands for "Low-density lipoprotein", transports cholesterol particles throughout the body and can build up in the walls of the arteries, making them harder and narrower. Lifestyle factors such as obesity, inactivity and unhealthy diet contribute to high cholesterol and low HDL cholesterol (good cholesterol). Some people, however, have a genetic predisposition that can keep cells from removing LDL cholesterol effectively from their blood or may cause the liver to produce too much of this cholesterol.

Those whose occupations involved either a high level of cognitive complexity or who engage in tasks that require high levels of alertness for safety reasons, may find that intermittent fasting interferes with their alertness in a way that impedes proper and safe performance during their occupations. Similar symptoms may include fatigue, dizziness and difficulty concentrating; a predictable consequence of the body absorbing subnormal levels of nutrients, even if the end results may be positive. Disrupted sleep cycles sometimes associated with intermittent fasting may only compound these side effects, as it may decrease the amount of REM sleep you are able to get, which is essential for memory, learning capacity and mood. Since fasting, like exercise, is a form of stress on the body (although it is a good form of stress, known as eustress, when conducted properly), one ought to expect higher than normal cortisol levels. Cortisol is the body's stress hormone and may further compound the psychological and emotional difficulty of navigating daily occupational and social tasks and concerns.

# Dos and Don'ts of Intermittent Fasting

## Questionable forms of fasting

Let us review some fasting protocols which, although popular, may not necessarily be healthy. Although at least some of these forms of fasting may yield benefits to some, there are notable risks involved and health professionals tend not to recommend them.

## The 48-Hour Fast

While most of the fasting protocols we have looked up allow some degree of food consumption even on fasting days, some people prefer more extreme 48-hour fasts. This protocol commonly accompanies intermittent fasting and it does have some benefits, but due to its extreme nature, it does have some drawbacks as well and these should be carefully noted prior to pursuing. Simply put, this regimen entails taking a full, two-day break from any food consumption whatsoever, and is commonly accomplished by eating nothing after dinner on the first day and not eating again until the third day. This is not a dry fast, so it is permissible to drink zero-calorie fluids like water, tea and black coffee. As with any fast, especially longer ones, it is important to drink plenty of fluids to prevent the dehydration that accompanies such fasts as a danger. Breaking this fast should be conducted gradually to avoid diarrhea, bloating and nausea through gut overstimulation, and the first post-fast meal should be a light snack like a couple handfuls of almonds followed by another small meal 1-2 hours after (Preiato, 2019).

Those who practice this kind of fast typically conduct it 1-2 times a month, as spacing out these fasts in such a way increases the benefits. As usual, it is important to refrain from eating unusually high amounts of high-calorie foods on non-fasting days, in order to prevent offsetting these benefits (Preiato, 2019). This form of fasting is not suitable for everyone, however, and it is probably better to stick with some of the other more moderate forms of intermittent fasting that we have discussed. If you do choose this form of fasting, it is best to first see if you can tolerate shorter fasts like alternate-day methods or the 16:8 protocol prior to attempting this more rigorous form of fasting.

Animal studies suggest that this form of fasting may improve cellular repair, which is the body's method of replenishing cells and thereby slowing aging, delaying tissue aging and preventing disease. Some research has likewise suggested that this method may reduce or prevent chronic inflammation, which can result in rheumatoid arthritis, cancer and heart disease. More specifically, fasting for more than 24 hours may reduce oxidative stress in the body's cells, which can lower inflammation (Preiato, 2019). As with some of the other forms of intermittent fasting we have discussed, this method may also improve insulin sensitivity and decrease insulin levels and blood sugar levels, as forms of fasting that exceed 24 hours deplete glycogen and are very effective at causing the body to burn fat for energy. One study in particular found that 10 individuals with type 2 diabetes who engaged in 12-72 hour fasting decreased blood sugar levels by up to 20 percent after only a single fasting regimen (Preiato, 2019).

While research on other forms of intermittent fasting demonstrate their efficacy in weight loss, there is not much research on 48-hour fasts in particular. Nevertheless, the fact that a regimen of 1-2 48-hour fasts per month can reduce calorie intake by up to 8,000 calories a month suggests that such benefits are plausible. Risks associated with this form of fasting are similar to those of more moderate forms, but they are amplified due to the longer duration. Severe hunger, insomnia, fatigue and dizziness ought to be expected among most of those who engage in this form of fasting. After 24 hours of fasting, the body will begin to burn fat for energy causing feelings of extreme sluggishness and fatigue, contributing dramatically to the difficulty of this regimen (Preiato, 2019).

Fasting for 48 hours should not be practiced by individuals with type 1 diabetes, people who are underweight or have a history of eating disorders, those with low blood pressure, or women who are pregnant, breastfeeding or trying to conceive. People taking certain medications such as blood thinners, insulin, NSAIDS or medication for blood pressure, should also refrain from this form of fasting. Fasting for greater than 24 hours is best done with potassium, calcium, magnesium and sodium supplements, as these essential electrolytes will quickly vanish with these more extreme forms of fasting. Drinking water with a small amount of either salt or electrolyte tablets can assist in this respect. Black coffee and green tea can help reduce hunger levels and flavored, non-calorie sparkling water can assist a great deal with hydration.

## What Is Water Fasting?

Water fasting is a particularly rigorous form of fasting that involves consuming nothing but water. Research shows that water fasting may lower the risk of certain chronic diseases such as diabetes, certain cancers and heart disease. It may also stimulate autophagy, which helps the body break down and recycle older components of your body's cells (Raman, 2019). Some of these older parts of these cells can be potentially dangerous, which may contribute to its protective health effect. Indeed, most of those who conduct water fasts are attempting to improve their health, prepare for a medical procedure, or sometimes, for spiritual or religious reasons.

Unfortunately, this particular form of fasting is not very well-studied at this time. The human and animal studies that have been conducted on this form of fasting, however, do suggest that it is capable of producing health effects. On the other hand, water fasting has been shown to be associated with certain health risks, some of which can be quite serious. Most water fasts last between 24 and 72 hours, and you should not continue a water fast longer than this apart from medical supervision. Most of those who engage in water fasting drink around 3 liters of water per day during the fast. Some popular contemporary diets and detoxing procedures are modeled after the water fast. The lemon detox cleanse is one of the more popular examples of this, which allows you to drink a mixture of water, lemon juice, maple syrup and cayenne pepper several times per day for up to a week (Raman, 2019).

As with other forms of fasting, pregnant women, children, older adults, individuals with eating disorders or chronic diseases (especially diabetes and gout) should avoid water fasting. Those who are new to water fasting ought to spend 3-4 days preparing the body for this protocol, preferably by eating smaller portions at each meal or fasting for part of each day in the days leading up to the beginning of the fast. Those who engage in this particularly extreme form of fasting may be even more susceptible than those who engage in the other forms of intermittent fasting to side effects such as weakness and dizziness.

For this reason, those operating heavy machinery or driving ought to avoid this form of fasting during these activities. Those who engage in water fasting may likewise be more susceptible to binging on a big meal following the fast, which can offset any benefits gained, and may likewise engage in other problematic symptoms. Breaking this fast ought to be done with either a smoothie or smaller meals, and you can thereafter continue with gradually introducing larger and larger meals throughout the day to the extent that you are comfortable. It is especially important to be mindful of eating habits during the post-fasting phase of these longer and more extreme fasts, since a potentially fatal condition known as refeeding syndrome may result if conducted improperly, which results when the body undergoes unusually rapid fluctuations in fluid and electrolyte levels.

## The Risk of Refeeding Syndrome

Some people are at greater risk of refeeding syndrome than others. Those who have experienced unexplained weight loss in the last six months totaling an amount greater than 10 percent of their total body weight, those whose body mass index (BMI) is less than 18.5, those who have consumed nothing but water for five or more days, those who either suffer from alcoholism or have a history of alcoholism, those whose blood work shows abnormally low levels of potassium, magnesium, calcium or phosphorus, those who have anorexia, or those who are undergoing chemotherapy, taking antacids, diuretics or insulin, are at statistically higher risk of this syndrome (Olsen, 2020). Those who are in the midst of breaking an unusually long fast are advised to do so with a meal that is low in carbohydrates and high in fat. Avoid sugary meals that increase insulin. If you are engaging in a water fast, drink 1 cup of bone breath every two or three days during this fast. Make sure to remain hydrated during your fast; mineral water may be especially helpful with this and supplementing it with a pinch of natural salt can be helpful as well.

Although refeeding syndrome is very rare, it is very serious when it does occur, and important steps must be taken in order to avoid it. Important clinical markers of this syndrome involve low blood serum levels of calcium, potassium and magnesium, and the symptoms, which usually appear between two and four days after the start of refeeding, can include heart rhythm abnormalities, confusion, fatigue, seizures, elevated blood pressure, weakness, breathing problems, cardiac arrest, convulsions, coma and death (Olsen, 2020). The syndrome was first described among severely malnourished Japanese prisoners held in war during World War II, and is sometimes observed in those with anorexia or among recovering alcoholics. These symptoms surface when insulin and counter-regulatory hormones such as noradrenaline and cortisol are abruptly reactivated, which causes a major movement of calcium, magnesium, phosphorus and potassium into our cells. Such depletion of our body stores can be excessive enough to leave us with too few ions in our blood, which can lead to the aforementioned symptoms (Olsen, 2020).

## The Benefits of Autophagy

During autophagy, older parts of the cells are broken down and recycled, which research suggests may protect against diseases like cancer, heart disease and Alzheimer's Disease. Recycling these cellular components may protect damaged parts of cells from accumulating, which protects against the growth of cancer cells, with animal research suggesting that water fasting may suppress the impact of genes that contribute to cancer growth and may also improve the effects of chemotherapy treatment. Animal studies likewise suggest that autophagy may help extend the organism's life span. Nevertheless, because few human studies have been conducted on the health impact of autophagy, processes that promote the process cannot be uncritically recommended as healthy. Some of the research that has been conducted on humans, however, may help individuals with high blood pressure lower their blood pressure. One study found that 68 individuals who suffered from borderline high blood pressure water fasted for nearly 14 days under medical supervision, resulting in the blood pressure of 82 percent of the participants dropping to healthy levels or lower (Raman, 2019).

Another study included 174 individuals with high blood pressure who water-fasted for an average of 10-11 days, resulting in blood pressure drops among 90 percent of the participants to much healthier levels (Raman, 2019). These particular examples of water fasts are quite extreme, however, and no human studies have investigated the link between short-term water fasts and blood pressure. Yet another study of 30 healthy adults who followed a water fast for 24 hours found much lower blood levels of triglycerides and cholesterol, both of which are significant risk factors for heart disease. Animal studies have likewise found that water fasting may protect the heart against damage resulting from the presence of free radicals; unstable molecules that can damage parts of the cells and are known to play an important role in many dangerous chronic diseases.

As with other forms of intermittent fasting we have discussed, water fasting may improve the body's sensitivity to both insulin and leptin, increasing the effectiveness of these hormones, both of which are important mechanisms of regulating the body's metabolism. Increased sensitivity to insulin means that your body is able to more effectively reduce blood sugar levels and also assists in storing the body's nutrients. Leptin, which helps the body feel full, may assist in

45

protecting against overeating by processing hunger signals, lowering the individual's risk of obesity (Raman, 2019).

Unfortunately, despite the potential for health benefits, much of the weight lost from this protocol can include water, carbs and muscle mass, rather than only the intended weight loss of unwanted fat. Ironically, water fasts may increase the risk of dehydration, since 20-30 percent of daily water intake comes from foods, and maintaining ordinary water consumption (as opposed to increasing it as necessary) may result in suboptimal water consumption. Those who engage in water fasts must therefore ensure that they make up for the water ordinarily acquired through food consumption by drinking more than they otherwise would. Dehydration can be quite serious, resulting in constipation, nausea, dizziness, headaches and low blood pressure (Raman, 2019). These symptoms may quite profoundly affect workplace productivity. Those susceptible to orthostatic hypotension may want to avoid water fasting, since it is a common symptom of the protocol. This is simply a fancy term for a drop in blood pressure that occurs when you stand up suddenly, which results in the individual feeling dizzy and lightheaded, and can increase your risk of fainting. It goes without saying that it is therefore unwise to undergo this fasting protocol when engaged in an occupation that involves operating heavy machinery or driving.

Since water fasting may increase uric acid production, those with gout may experience unusually severe symptoms. Those with diabetes should avoid water fasting or consult with a physician before attempting it, and, as with forms of intermittent fasting, those with eating disorders or who are susceptible to disordered patterns ought to consult with a physician before attempting this procedure (Raman, 2019). Despite the health benefits which may accrue from water fasting, those interested in losing weight through caloric restriction may be better off resorting to other forms of fasting, such as intermittent fasting and alternate day fasting, which are likely more effective, and certainly far safer. These other forms of fasting are safer and can also be followed with much longer periods, providing the benefits of weight loss with decreased risk of nutritional deficiencies.

## Understanding Dry Fasting

Despite the demonstrable benefits of various intermittent fasting methods, some individuals take a more extreme approach to intake restriction that goes beyond mere caloric restriction, in the form of "dry fasting." Dry fasting entails abstaining, not only from food and non-caloric liquids, but from all liquids altogether. This protocol can be dangerous, since you run the risk of several complications, most obviously, dehydration. In addition to its dangers, there is not enough research on the benefits of dry fasting to recommend it, especially in light of the greater amount of research done on safer forms of fasting, and the benefits found in such research.

Advocates of dry fasting state that it is a more effective means of weight loss than ordinary fasting due to the extreme nature of the caloric restriction undertaken. A 2013 study in the Journal of Human Nutrition and Dietetics examined the effects of such fasting among Muslims during Ramadan, who do not eat or drink at all from sunrise to sunset. Of the 240 healthy adults who fasted for at least 20 days, almost all of them have experienced a sharp drop in body weight and BMI following the experience. Of course, those engaging in this dry fasting were engaging in intermittent fasting, whose benefits are demonstrable and well-known, and abstaining from drinking during this period may or may not have contributed to the weight loss (at any rate, it does not appear to have impeded it). Nevertheless, it is unclear whether these results can be consistently replicated and whether their safety can be demonstrated.

Some advocates of dry fasting claim that this procedure strengthens the body's immune system by "resetting" the system and removing the body's damaged cells, allowing the body to replace it with new ones. There certainly is evidence that limiting calories does have this impact on inflammation, but it has not been scientifically demonstrated that dry fasting has this impact. One paper, however, published in 2012 in Nutrition Research measured proinflammatory cytokines in 50 healthy adults one week prior to Ramadan, and then again during the third week and one month after their dry fasting during Ramadan. According to the researchers, the proinflammatory cytokines of the participants were indeed lowest during the third week of dry fasting, suggesting that it may indeed have such anti-inflammatory benefits.

Some advocates of dry fasting insist that it can do the same. Indeed, advocates of dry fasting who argue that it can slow down skin aging may point to a 2018 study in Cell Metabolism, which found that calorie restriction reduced biomarkers of aging in 53 young, healthy adults. Nevertheless, as with many of these studies, such benefits are not restricted to (or even necessarily increased by) dry fasting, but appear to the consequence simply of intermittent fasting, even when done alongside liquid consumption. This would certainly be surprising, since it is known that water intake promotes healthy skin, possibly due to its allegedly healthy impact on the immune system (Butler, 2019).

Although some research suggests that such fasting protocols may improve wound healing, there is conflicting evidence on this. A 2019 review in Nutrients states that increased immune activity resulting from fasting assists in wound healing. Prior to this, a 2011 animal study found similar effects on mice when they were subjected to repeated, temporary fasts. Nevertheless, a 2012 animal study in Age found that similar calorie restriction protocols impaired the ability of rats to heal their wounds. At this time, there is not enough evidence to definitively come to one conclusion or the other (Butler, 2019).

Some of the alleged benefits of dry fasting are purely subjective and personal, which make them hard to dispute. For example, those who use the practice for spiritual and religious purposes relate that it enhances their faith, improves their gratitude, and provides them greater opportunity for prayer. Intriguingly enough, however, these alleged benefits are not reported solely by Muslims or by any other one religious faith but are instead reported by all of those who participate in the practice, regardless of whether or not they report a specific religious or spiritual alignment.

Unfortunately, only the kind of intermittent dry fasting conducted by Muslims during Ramadan have been examined with any degree of rigor and more research is needed to get a better sense of how intermittent dry fasting compares with other forms of fasting. One review published in 2019, in Eastern Mediterranean Health Journal, found that the intermittent dry fasting practiced by Muslims during Ramadan has similar effects to other forms of intermittent fasting that do not restrict all liquid intake. Importantly, if dry fasting is something that you intend to practice, it is necessary to be cognizant of health risks (Butler, 2019).

Dry fasting has potential side effects that are comparable to other forms of intermittent fasting, but at least some of these side effects may be more substantial. For example, persistent hunger is something that anyone who is fasting ought to expect to struggle with, but this subjective side effect will be more pronounced during intermittent dry fasting, since water tends to increase satiety or help you feel full. Lacking water will mean that your body has even less fuel than it does with other forms of intermittent fasting, and this may cause you to feel even more tired than you would while engaging in other forms of intermittent fasting. As with other forms of intermittent fasting, you will experience irritability, nutrition deficiencies, headaches and poor focus if you engage in dry fasting. Be advised that eliminating all fluid intake will cause you to urinate less frequently, and it will cause your urine to become dark and foul-smelling (Butler, 2019).

The dramatically increased risk of dehydration causes this method to pose much higher risk than other forms of intermittent fasting. Such dehydration may result in electrolyte imbalances and can cause dangerously low blood pressure. Lack of fluids can also lead to urinary and kidney problems, such as kidney stones and urinary tract infections. Although the low blood sugar associated with intermittent fasting may always increase the risk of fainting, the combination of this with dehydration can further increase this risk. Positive and negative effects of dry fasting vary from one individual to the next, and depend upon factors such as age, daily activity level, overall health and how often you fast.

## Juice Fasting

As we have seen, it is important to be selective when determining what sorts of liquids you choose to incorporate into your fasting regimen. Water is always essential (except for those dry fasting), and unsweetened tea and coffee are also popular options, but in recent years, juice fasting has increased in popularity. As the name suggests, this protocol entails drinking only liquids, although some of those who engage in juice fasting do incorporate water, tea and other clear liquids as well. Also known as juice cleansing, those who choose this option are attempting to increase the amount of nutrients in their bodies in addition to merely attempting to lose weight. Other alleged benefits include boosting the immune system and removing toxins from the body.

Juice fasting entails drinking liquid extracts from both whole fruits and vegetables and those who prefer this method of fasting say that they enjoy the benefits of the nutrients of these substances while giving their digestive systems a rest from the harsh (if necessary) presence of fiber, which can be rough on those with digestive system issues.

Joe Cross famously engaged in a particularly extreme juice fast, which he discusses in his documentary *Fat, Sick and Nearly Dead*, during which he claims to have lost 100 pounds on a 60-day juice fast. In his New York Times best-selling book, *The Reboot with Joe Juice Diet*, he articulates a juice fast protocol that includes 80 percent vegetables and 20 percent fruits. Make sure that your juices are diverse in order to guarantee that you get all of your required nutrients. "Green" juices can be a helpful way of ensuring that you get all of your vegetables in addition to the fruits and can contain some (but not too much) spinach, kale, broccoli, celery or romaine lettuce, with apples and pears to add some sweetness. Ginger, carrots, beets, and sweet potatoes can also make a nice addition.

Although it is certainly good to include vegetables in your juice, avoid juices that have a great deal of certain kinds of green leafy vegetables like spinach or kale. Such vegetables contain goitrogen, which can adversely impact your body's absorption of iodine leading to slowed thyroid function. Side effects from this method of fasting may include diarrhea, dizziness, constipation or fatigue. More severe side effects may include vomiting, fainting, severe diarrhea, dizziness or low blood pressure.

It ought to be noted that most doctors do not recommend this method of fasting since the lack of protein may lead to muscle atrophy. Not only can this account for part of the weight loss, but the amount of sugar juices tend to contain can lead to unwanted weight gain, in addition to the blood sugar swings associated with high levels of sugar consumption. Indeed, one of the dangers of the juice fast is that once the fast itself is ended, and the ordinary diet resumes, you may see your progress lost when the previously lost weight is regained.

Be sure to be careful about consuming raw, unpasteurized juices, especially if you are an older adult, pregnant, a young child or suffer from a compromised immune system. As always, wash fruits and vegetables if you are making your own smoothie to eliminate any unwanted bacteria, and only juice which you intend to consume in one sitting since fresh juices can quickly become not-so-fresh and generate this unwanted bacteria before long. If you do not consume all of the contents in one sitting, store it in a clean, airtight container and ensure it is adequately refrigerated. If you have not finished consuming it within 24 hours, the contents should be discarded.

One of the major problems with juice-related fasting is that those who participate in it may not feel adequately full, and this may tempt the faster to break their fast, especially through consumption of unhealthy foods. This is not only because liquid meals tend to be less filling than meals that consist of solid food, especially when these meals are high in carbohydrates, but also because juice fasting typically lacks fiber and protein, both of which contribute to a feeling of fullness you normally (and ideally) enjoy after a meal (Elliott, 2016). Indeed, apart from typically lacking protein, the juicing process eliminates what fiber you would normally obtain from fruit consumption. For example, in one study, 20 adults of normal weight and 20 adults who were overweight were each given 300 calories worth of fruit, consisting of apple sauce, an apple or apple juice.

Those who drank the apple juice did not feel as full as those who had consumed solid foods and ended up hungry earlier than the others. It may be preferable, therefore, provided you have a healthy gastrointestinal system, that you choose a form of intermittent fasting that allows you to consume protein and fiber due to their appetite-reducing properties. For example, protein increases the levels of hormones that help you feel full, assisting in appetite regulation while fiber helps reduce appetite by slowing down the rate at which your stomach empties itself of food and increases the time it takes for digestion to occur (Elliott, 2016). Lacking these substances in your intermittent fasting regimen can make your time a great deal more difficult. Fiber is important, not only for feeling full, but for other dietary reasons as well. It helps beneficial bacteria thrive in your digestive system, reduces constipation in some individuals and may also reduce your risk of heart disease, diabetes and obesity. Therefore, as long as you have a healthy digestive system that can tolerate adequate fiber intake, it may be preferable to choose another form of intermittent fasting (Elliott, 2016).

In addition to lacking fiber and protein, adopting a juice fast may be less than ideal due to the deficiency of vitamin D, iron, calcium, zinc, vitamin B12 and omega-3 fatty acids that can result from it. One of the reasons for the danger of vitamin deficiency during a juice fast has to do with the low levels of fat in fruits, which is required for the absorption of fat-soluble vitamins such as A, D, E and K. The oxalate in greens such as spinach, beet greens and turnip greens that are oftentimes added to juices may also impede absorption of important nutrients. Despite the avowed benefits from its advocates of immune system boosting, low levels of zinc and iron may impede immune system function, leading to increased risk of infection (Elliott, 2016).

## Avoiding dehydration

As with everything else, when it comes to fasting, there is a right and a wrong way to do it. Conducted in moderation and according to a scientifically validated protocol, it can provide tremendous health benefits, but done carelessly or in excess, it can be quite dangerous. Most of the regimens that we have looked up recommend short fasting periods of between 8-24 hours. Nevertheless, some of our more Herculean friends conduct fasts between 48 and 72 hours. Fasting for longer than this, if not done carefully and with a great deal of precision, can begin to cause various difficulties and health problems, such as irritability, hunger, lack of energy, fainting, difficulty concentrating and dehydration. Avoiding dehydration is one of the most important elements of safe fasting, as we have seen. It becomes a risk even during intermittent fasting and is increased as a risk with a form of periodic fasting known as water fasting. This risk becomes an even greater risk yet during forms of fasting that prohibit liquid consumption such as dry fasting.

Dehydration ultimately occurs when you lose more fluid than you take in, leading to your body eventually not having enough water or other fluids to function normally. Failure to replace these lost fluids can lead to dehydration, which can be especially dangerous, and even life-threatening, to young children or older adults. In young children, the most common symptom is severe diarrhea and vomiting. Other signs of dehydration in young children may include an absence of tears when crying, dry mouth and tongue, no wet diapers for three hours, irritability, or sunken soft spot on the top of the infant's skull.

Those who are elderly tend to naturally have lower levels of water in their bodies and may have either conditions or have to take medication that may further increase the risk of dehydration. Elderly individuals who choose to engage in fasting ought to therefore be especially diligent that they remain adequately hydrated. Indeed, older adults tend to exhibit a lower fluid reserve, leading to difficulties conserving water. The individual's sense of thirst may also become less acute, and these problems may be further compounded by chronic illnesses more commonly associated with old age, such as dementia, especially when associated with the use of the aforementioned medications that may contribute to increased urination.

In adults, it tends to be characterized by extreme thirst, less frequent urination, darker-colored urine, fatigue, confusion, and dizziness. It is important to contact a doctor if you have had diarrhea for 24 hours or more, cannot keep down fluids, suffer from bloody or black stool or have been irritable, disoriented or unusually sleepy. Dehydration is sometimes the result of simply not drinking enough water but may also result from fever. In general, the higher the fever, the greater the risk of dehydration. Failure to replace fluids in the midst of excessive sweating, whether as the result of hot, humid weather or vigorous activity, can also result in dehydration. Those with certain medical conditions like uncontrolled diabetes, can lead to increased urination that can eventually result in dehydration. This is also true of certain medications, such as blood pressure medications or diuretics.

Failing to drink enough fluids, especially when working vigorously in the hot, humid weather, can lead to heat injury. Some forms of heat injury, such as mild heat cramps, can be easily remedied. Heat exhaustion is more serious, however, and heatstroke can be potentially life-threatening. Prolonged bouts of dehydration, if sufficiently severe, can even lead to outright kidney failure. Failure to replenish electrolytes such as potassium and sodium can likewise contribute to seizures because they impede the ability of the body to carry electrical signals from cell to cell. Interfering with normal electrical messages in such a way can lead to involuntary muscle contractions and even to fainting. Worse yet, low blood volume shock, also known as hypovolemic shock, may set in once low blood volume causes a drop in blood pressure, thus causing a drop in the amount of oxygen in the body. This is one of the most serious consequences of more severe dehydration and can be life-threatening.

While dehydration is certainly no joke, its symptoms are usually relatively mild, and produce enough discomfort that most individuals will spontaneously drink the amount of water necessary to remedy them. These milder symptoms can result in dry mouth, fatigue, thirst and headaches. Although mild to moderate hydration is usually reversible by drinking more fluids, severe dehydration requires immediate medical treatment. For this reason, many of those who fast drink 8.5 to 13 cups of water over the course of the day, although you should always drink whatever amount you feel your body needs, as long as it is within a safe range. How much fluid you require will vary based on the individual, but most health authorities recommend the 8x8 rule. This recommendation includes eight 8-ounce glasses of fluid (preferably water) every day. It is especially important to be mindful of the body's fluid requirements while fasting, since you get around 20-30 percent of fluid from food, increasing the risk of dehydration while fasting.

## Starting Slow

Although individuals seeking to fast for more than 72 hours may pursue such a regimen under medical supervision, in general, it is better to stick with shorter fasting periods of up to 24 hours, especially if you are only just beginning. Those who are new to fasting may want to begin with the 5:2 diet, since it allows you to consume up to 25% of caloric requirements on fasting days. This ensures that you are restricting caloric intake to a degree that produces the intended effects of fasting, without so depriving you of nutrients that you suffer from some of the aforementioned difficulties associated with more rigorous fasting regimens.

Although you might still feel faint, hungry and have some difficulty concentrating at times, being able to consume up to a quarter of daily caloric requirements will certainly mitigate these effects. Although some might be concerned that this degree of permissiveness might impede the intended weight loss effects of fasting, allowing up to a quarter of daily caloric intake might actually be more effective than other more extreme forms of fasting, especially for beginners, because it will make the regimen more tolerable and sustainable and you will feel less tempted to binge or feast, offsetting whatever gains you may have acquired during the period. Indeed, when you break your fast, it is not recommended to do so with a feast, as this may defeat the whole purpose of the fasting regimen, and you may end up taking two steps forward only to then take two steps backwards.

Eating too large a meal on the day following your fast may leave you feeling tired and bloated. Instead of binging, simply resume your ordinary eating schedule and habits (provided they are healthy; if they are not, change your regular eating habits so that they are). It is especially important to be very mindful of returning to ordinary eating patterns after fasting, because such caloric restriction can tempt you a great deal to "feast" and eat more than you would ordinarily. Research shows that going too long without eating, or going too long without eating a "normal" amount, can tempt you to gorge, which will cause you to feel less satisfied after you have eaten, and will cause you to continue to eat before your body knows that you have already had enough.

Apart from these physical requirements, much of the battle in conducting a successful fast is psychological. Fasting can be quite difficult, especially for those who lack a means of distracting themselves and end up bored and hungry enough to be tempted by tasty morsels. An idle stomach is the devil's plaything and making sure you remain occupied with something productive or entertaining is a great way of staving off the temptation to break your fast prematurely. Walking and meditating are both helpful ways of keeping yourself on the straight path, and in fact, there is actually a Sutta dedicated specifically to walking meditation in the ancient Buddhist Pali Canon that not only provides the helpful distractions of walking and meditating, but also advocates the use of mindfulness during this period of walking / meditating, which is itself an effective way of dealing with psychological discomfort in general. The "Cankama Sutta" is quite short, especially compared with many other writings in the Pali Canon, and states in its entirety:

"Monks, there are these five benefits of walking up & down [walking a prescribed path]. What five?

One is fit for long journeys; one is fit for striving; one has little disease; that which is eaten, drunk, chewed, tasted, goes through proper digestion; the composure attained by walking up & down is long-lasting.

These, monks, are the five benefits of walking up & down."

In this Sutta, we find that walking, meditating and catering to digestive health are all addressed in one fell swoop! It is important to not engage in activity that is too strenuous, however, and pursuing an engaging activity that does not burn too much energy, such as reading a book, is recommended. That said, it is important to keep any exercise you engage in mild when fasting. Although some find that they are able to effectively maintain periods of regular exercise while fasting, low-intensity exercises are recommended for those who are new to the practice. This might include housework, gentle stretching or yoga. Some may struggle even during these mild exercises, which is okay. If you find that you are struggling, rest and do not strain yourself.

Although some degree of discomfort, physical and psychological, is predictable and perhaps even inevitable (fatigue, irritability and hunger), feeling "unwell" is a major red flag, and if you ever began to feel genuinely sick rather than just mildly uncomfortable, you should resume your ordinary, healthy diet and consult with a physician before continuing to fast. This is especially true if you begin to experience tiredness, weakness or fatigue that is severe enough to prevent you from carrying out your ordinary, daily tasks, or if you begin to experience feelings of sickness and discomfort that are unusual.

When it comes to fasting, eating properly on non-fasting days is just as important as not eating on fasting days. Make sure that you consume enough protein when you do eat, in order to avoid losing muscle you want to keep along with the fat you are trying to lose. If you are undergoing a period of intermittent fasting that allows you to eat small amounts on fasting days, make sure you snack on protein on those days as well. Research suggests that consuming even 30% of a meal's calories from protein can majorly reduce feelings of hunger and make fasting that much more bearable. Eating whole foods on non-fasting days (and on fasting days where the protocol permits it) can likewise reduce risk of cancer, heart disease and other chronic illnesses. Whole foods include fish, meat, eggs, fruits, vegetables and legumes (if you want to kill two birds with one stone, meat, fish and eggs are whole foods that contain a great deal of protein).

Consuming healthy supplements is always recommended for those engaging in fasting protocols. This is because consuming fewer calories makes it more difficult to meet daily nutritional needs. Since those engaging in weight loss diets are more likely to be deficient in essential nutrients like calcium, iron and vitamin B12, supplements containing these nutrients are especially recommended. Although your best bet is always to acquire your nutrients from whole foods when possible, multivitamins that cater to all your nutritional needs are especially recommended wherever a caloric deficit may interfere with meeting them in a healthy way.

## Eat Slowly!

Those who fast, especially those who engage in some of the more extreme forms of fasting, may be susceptible to a behavioral pattern with which most Americans already struggle: The tendency to eat too quickly. The problem with this is that those who eat too quickly will take in too many calories before the body knows that it has already taken in enough calories. This is because it takes about 20 minutes from the time you begin eating for your brain to generate signals associated with feeling full, and it is for this reason that it is important to eat slowly enough to provide the amount of time necessary to signal to the brain that you are full. This allows you to stop eating prior to consuming more calories than are necessary or healthy. This is especially important when eating dessert, where calories are often proportionately more abundant than they might be during the main course. Those who enjoy dessert are therefore urged to take one, reasonably sized bite at a time and slowly enjoy and savor the experience rather than quickly eating the entire portion without restraint.

Indeed, research shows that overweight men and women consume fewer calories when they slow their pace of eating. Those who have had gastric bypass operations are especially urged to eat more slowly, since those who fail to do so, according to research, are less successful at losing weight than other patients. Besides, those who eat more quickly are less likely to enjoy their meal. Those with more of a "type A" temperament may want to put on some relaxing music and light some candles in order to assist in the sort of relaxation that will assist with this process. Although experts recommend against allowing more than 4 hours to pass between each meal, this is not always possible within the context of fasting. Therefore, the hungry dieter who is about to break his or her fast must be especially careful to eat slowly. Drinking a large glass of water and waiting for a bit after the first serving, before helping yourself to another serving, may help you feel fuller before you eat more calories than are necessary.

Importantly, eating too quickly can have very negative health consequences. Research shows that those who eat more slowly are less likely to become obese and less likely to develop metabolic syndrome, which is a complex of health problems that increases the risk of other serious health problems such as diabetes, stroke, heart disease, high blood sugar, high blood pressure and low HDL cholesterol. In addition to eating more slowly, it is important to take more time to chew your food adequately. Healthy eating, involving whole grains, fruits and vegetables, supplemented with a healthy amount of exercise, also reduces the risk of developing metabolic syndrome.

## Eat in Moderation!

The temptation of eating too much, and the problems associated with this practice, of course, go hand in hand with eating too quickly. Eating too quickly causes the digestive system to work much harder than it needs to, predictably leads to an upset stomach, and can cause a spike in blood sugar, along with feelings of lethargy. Importantly, although many of us might intuitively associate overeating with consumption of junk food, it is actually possible to eat too much healthy food. What exactly constitutes overeating depends a great deal on the individual and has a lot to do with how much your body is able to handle at any given time. Relevant variables include age, height, amount of exercise, sleeping patterns and medical problems you may have. Those who experience difficulty with keeping note of how much they eat, and when they eat, may benefit from food journals, mindfulness, intuitive eating and portion control. This will help them develop strategies necessary in determining when your body is full and when it is hungry due to lack of adequate nutrients.

It is important to listen to your body during this process. Those who may experience a kind of hot flash in mid-bite may indicate that you have overeaten. This is because this spike in body temperature is an indication that your body is in the process of digesting what it has already eaten, and it may be beneficial to take a break from eating to allow the feeling of fullness following this digestive process to emerge. Taking such breaks will help alleviate feelings of bloating or discomfort, and if taking such breaks is your only way of alleviating discomfort which you are already experiencing during food consumption, it is likely that you are eating too much. More intuitively, if you are put off by eating what is left on your plate, this is a telltale sign that your brain already knows that your body is full, and you should not force yourself to consume more food.

The spikes in blood sugar levels resulting from overeating ends up generating more insulin than is ordinary or necessary to keep blood sugar levels in a healthy range, which can lead to headaches, thirst, lethargy and fatigue. This can be associated with the storing of excess blood sugar and calories, which can lead to unhealthy weight gain. Some of these symptoms of physical discomfort are the consequences of your digestive organ swelling and bloating, which can lead to nausea and acid reflux.

The mind and the body are intimately intertwined, since the brain produces the mind, and the brain is part of the body. It should therefore come as no surprise that overeating, as with any unhealthy physical activities, can adversely affect the brain, and therefore, the mind. Indeed, research suggests that overeating, especially where this involves consumption of foods high in fat and sugar for an extended period, can adversely impact cognitive function, leading to symptoms such as memory loss and impaired judgment. These unfortunate behavioral and psychological side effects have been associated with increased white matter in the brain, which is normally associated with the elderly.

Those who struggle with overeating ought to drink the recommended six to eight glasses of water per day in order to keep hydrated and help the body digest. This will also help detoxify the system from excessive sodium intake. Of course, those who are fasting may need to drink more than this recommended standard amount of water, since much of the water acquired throughout the day comes from our ordinary food intake rather than the consumption of liquid. Although intense exercise is not recommended after you have eaten, especially in the event of a large meal, going for a light walk or practicing yoga can assist in healthier digestion, and regular exercise spaced out appropriately between meals can jumpstart the metabolism and help work off extra and unwanted calories.

## Avoid Excess Sugar

It is well-known, among both experts and laymen, that excessive sugar consumption is harmful to our health. It is especially important for those who are engaging in fasting to understand this, however, because there are several consequences of excess sugar intake that can make fasting more difficult and offset whatever benefits you may have gained. This becomes especially difficult in modern Western diets, where what we see on the shelves are loaded with added sweeteners even in items we might consider relatively innocuous, in addition to the more usual and well-known culprits, like candy, processed snack foods, canned food and soft drinks.

Since sugary foods and drinks have a ton of calories, those who are fasting would do well to avoid them as much as possible. These items not only add unwanted calories and the associated weight but very little nutritional benefit. When more sugar is consumed than is necessary, the body converts it into fatty acid and stores it in adipose fatty cells for future use, which tends to become visible on our bodies in the form of obesity.

Sugar also tends to interact with bacteria and produce acids in the mouth that damage tooth enamel, producing tooth decay. Sugar does not itself actually cause cavities, however, which are actually the waste product caused by sugar interacting with the surface of the teeth. In addition to watching what you eat, it is important to undergo regular dental cleanses. Various skin conditions such as skin dullness and rosacea may also be associated with excess sugar consumptions.

Those who are fasting are already craving food, and may be especially desirous of sugar, but the more sugar you consume, the more you crave it. There is controversy as to whether it is like being addicted to hard drugs, and it is not clear exactly how addictive sugar is, but such cravings are unhealthy for the ordinary person and especially disastrous for those trying to fast. One 2008 study published in the "Neuroscience & Biobehavioral Reviews" journal found that when given unlimited access to sugar, rats began to binge, exhibited withdrawal symptoms, and began to crave more sugar (Hebebrand et. al, 2014). Since those who are fasting may already be struggling with the temptation to binge, sugar can only exacerbate this problem and may make the process more difficult. Disturbingly, this study even found that excess sugar appeared to overlay in its causal mechanisms with other more devastating forms of substance abuse (Hebebrand et. al, 2014)

Diets high in sugar have also been linked with various forms of mental illness, such as depression. Sugar itself is considered inflammatory and releases the "feel-good" neurotransmitter known as dopamine, which may contribute to its addictive properties. Apart from being unhealthy in many other respects, diets high in starch and sugar are linked with inflammation at a much higher level than those rich in healthier foods such as vegetables and one protein. A great deal of high-quality research suggests that inflammation is a strong indicator of both depression and high stress levels, and anxiety, stress and depression may lead you to seek out sugary foods, since these produce the sort of "feel good" effect associated with dopamine. The ways in which these consumption habits may adversely impact your fasting regimen, therefore, have a strong psychological component rather than being linked purely to physiology. In addition to having far more calories than nutrients, sugar actually impedes your brain's capacity to know when you are full. This causes you to become more likely to overeat as a consequence of refined sugars and saturated fats interfering with the brain's ability to signal to the body that you have consumed adequate nutrition.

# What to Do If You Have Overeaten

The battle for the successful fasting regimen is as much a psychological one as it is physiological. Nobody is perfect, and we all make mistakes, and it should therefore come as no surprise that you may find that you have overeaten. If you have stumbled into this temptation, do not despair or feel guilty over having done so. The occasional mistake will not destroy your efforts, and too much guilt overeating habits can lead to unhealthy consumption behaviors, either through eating too much or excessive self-denial in the form of eating too little.

Before we look at some of the countermeasures for those who have already overeaten, a helpful way of preventing overeating in the first place is to meticulously plan your eating pattern for the entire week. Fasting is not something that ought to be done through improvisation and requires a great deal of foresight. Since our ancestors evolved in the midst of the danger of famine, impulse control when it comes to food is not necessarily something that we naturally excel at, and it is important to mobilize our higher-order cognitive faculties in order to guard against this otherwise natural temptation to immediately scarf down whatever appears appetizing. Make sure you choose meals that are low in calories, and prepare as many of these meals as you can in advance in order to avoid the frustration involved in having to prepare impromptu meals at the last minute and the temptation to have recourse to have less healthy instant-gratification in the form of something like fast food or vending machines that can result from this.

When you do it, it is often helpful to be "mindful" of your food consumption in the same way the ancient Buddhists were mindful. Allow yourself to be acutely conscious of the feel, texture and flavor of the food as you slowly chew and swallow the morsels in small bites. Contemplate how, when and where you prepared the food. If you did not prepare the food yourself, consider thinking about who grew it or who prepared it and how this was accomplished. As you slowly chew and contemplate the food, you give yourself more time to register what you have eaten and feel satisfied, which will give your brain enough time to signal to your body that you are full from adequate nutrition and prevent you from overeating again (Kubala, 2019). It takes the brain about 20 minutes to signal to the body that you are full and adequately fed, so if you eat an excessively large meal in 10 minutes, your brain will not be aware of this until it is too late. It is better to consume food with lots of fiber and protein, such as whole grains and vegetables during this process, since these are more conducive to feeling full. Avoid fatty meat, white bread or French fries, and replace them with whole grains and vegetables and you will feel full sooner.

If you do find that you have overeaten, there are healthy steps you can take to counteract its effects. A light walk can help stimulate digestion and even our blood sugar levels. A light bike ride may be helpful as well, but it is important not to workout too rigorously if you have overeaten, since this could send blood to your legs instead of stomach, which could slow digestion and have the opposite of its intended effect. Instead, it may help to take a casual ride or walk through a park or some other environment you find relaxing. Although intense exercise is recommended for getting rid of unwanted weight and calories, it is important to wait 3-4 hours before doing so in order to jumpstart your metabolism and prevent exercise. This will also control your hunger and help regulate your mood in a positive direction, which will protect against overeating in the future (Zelman, 2019).

Sip on a cup of water of about 8 ounces after a big meal in order to eliminate excess salt. This can prevent constipation. Drink water in moderation throughout the rest of the day to remain hydrated. Even if you choose not to exercise, avoid lying down so you can burn off some of those excess calories. Doing the dishes or some other necessary chore will help you to kill two birds with one stone, burning off some calories and accomplishing something you may have been putting off (Zelman, 2019). Lying down, on the other hand, can cause food to work its way back up when you have a full stomach, which can slow digestion and exacerbate the acid reflux that can sometimes result from overeating.

Avoid carbonated drinks since these can cause you to feel even more bloated than you already feel from the food you have consumed in excess. It also helps you give away any leftovers you may have from the meal. The reason for this is that holding on to the remaining food can trick your brain into thinking that you have not actually eaten enough even though you have actually eaten too much. This can cause you to eat even more and exercise less, which is the exact opposite of what is recommended after having overeaten. If you do decide to keep leftovers, divide them into single portions so that if you do decide to eat, you are not tempted to eat too much and make sure the remaining food is not high-calorie or sugary, since this can be especially counterproductive if you do decide to eat the remainders (Zelman, 2019).

If you find that you are frequently overeating, especially in spite of efforts to cease the behavior, it may be important to talk with a physician or mental health professional. Those who engage in binging habitually may suffer from a binge eating disorder, and this may be associated with feelings of self-loathing or despair after failures following repeated attempts to eat healthier. Over time, this can cause a great deal of damage to your body and your mind, so it is important to seek out the help of a doctor if you find yourself in such a situation or one similar to it.

## Handling Frustration

It is totally natural and predictable, whether you are only just beginning to fast for the first time, or whether you are a veteran faster, that you want to simply give up out of despair and discouragement. The degree and intensity to which this becomes a temptation has a great deal to do with the length of your fast and the type of fasting you are practicing, as well as many other factors, some physical and some psychological. Low energy, headaches and hunger can weigh heavily on the mind for anyone and it is important to arm yourself before you begin with ways to ensure you are encouraged even in the midst of difficulty. Of course, if you experience severe discomfort that feels abnormal or disabling, it is important to cease fasting and consult with a physician as quickly as possible.

As Dr. Gloriane points out, one of the main causes of abandoning your fast is plain and simple fear and other negative emotions. Food is not just about survival, as she points out, many people do not realize just how deep and profound a role fasting plays in our basic and most primitive psychological and emotional drives until they begin to fast for a first time. Food can come to focus as a surrogate for love or connection, a security blanket, a means of comfort, an occasion for celebration or a drug for relief or even as a means of dysfunctional soothing for serious mental health problems. Removing readily accessible food from our lives may deprive us of our largely unconscious means of self-soothing and self-medication and cause us to feel very vulnerable and exposed to psychological pain of which we had not even been conscious, or of which we had been only dimly aware. Indeed, the human brain makes countless decisions and is faced with innumerable impulses and thoughts each day, and you may be surprised to learn just how many of them have to do with food.

In light of these temptations, it is helpful to articulate to yourself some psychological correctives that can prevent you from succumbing to breaking your fast. First, remind yourself of why you chose to fast and focus on the benefits that will eventually accrue, and the happiness which those benefits will bring. Make sure to remove any tempting foods from your house so it is not possible for them to serve as occasions to temptation, and replace them with music, meditation, walks, reading and movies, or other helpful activities. Avoid the kitchen where possible and politely ask those around you to be discreet when eating food, especially if they are eating something unhealthy, sugary or laden with calories. If you are afraid of confrontation emerging from such incidents, it may be better to plan to be elsewhere and avoid such situations whenever possible. Be mindful of painful emotions and fears that crop up. Do not attempt to suppress them or judge them harshly, but simply allow yourself to be aware of them as they surface in your conscious mind and perhaps attempt to examine their basis through introspection.

Most people will find that, at bottom, these fears, insecurities and feelings of vulnerability have no basis in reality and will begin to dissipate in strength. In this respect, fasting can serve as a powerful psychological therapy rather than merely as a means of losing weight and looking or feeling better physically. You will find at the end of your fast that your feelings of attachment towards food may have dramatically decreased in strength, and may come to find that your relationship with yourself, both mind and body, has become much healthier in a way you had not expected from what you may have initially regarded as a purely physical endeavor.

# How To Break Your Fast

It is just as important to understand how to safely and effectively break or end a fast as it is to learn how to begin and endure it. Those who have fast for a great length of time will experience their body slow down its production of digestive enzymes, which may cause gastrointestinal distress and related discomfort once they resume normal food consumption. Such discomfort may include passing of undigested foods, gassiness, diarrhea or loose stools, bloating, and in severe cases, nausea and vomiting. Once you break your fast, food will tend to sit in your stomach for longer than normal, as the body does not have the relevant digestive enzymes and juices readily available to break them down as it had in the past. It can therefore take at least a few hours, and perhaps longer, for the body to resume its normal secretion of relevant chemicals to break down the food you have begun to consume normally again. Fasting more regularly and planning ideal foods for breaking the fast can help alleviate these symptoms to some degree. When you fast more regularly, the body becomes accustomed to this routine and does not cease production of digestive enzymes the way it might for those who abruptly fast out of nowhere.

Special care should be undertaken in ending the case for the first two months after you have begun fasting or whenever you choose to increase the duration of your fast. This is similarly true if you are fasting for unusually long durations when your last meal was high in carbohydrates or if you have begun to fast after a period of eating more than usual. When you do break your fast, avoid foods like nuts or nut butters, raw cruciferous vegetables, eggs, alcohol, dairy products or seeds and seed butters (Ramos 2020).

Six or so hours after ending the fast, however, should be enough time for you to resume ordinary food consumption. On the other hand, for those who tend to experience distress when breaking fasts, it is recommended to start off the break-fast well-hydrated and to consume chicken salad with leaf vegetables and cherry tomatoes. The best protein sources for breaking a fast are poultry or fish and these can be cooked in fat. Non-starchy vegetables that have been cooked in healthy fats, such as butter, ghee, coconut oil or avocado can be helpful (Ramos 2020).

Avoid alcohol after breaking a fast, especially when it comes to heavy consumption following a fast that has lasted more than a day. Binge drinking following such a fast can trigger alcoholic ketoacidosis, which can result in dangerously high levels of ketones in the blood. Symptoms of this disorder include vomiting and abdominal pain and are most common in those suffering from alcoholism who drink heavily after going days without eating (Ramos 2020).

While fasting, especially when done in moderation, is not likely to result in nutritional deficiency, some people choose to take various supplements in order to ensure that they are experiencing adequate vitamin and mineral intake. Nevertheless, it is important to understand which supplements are permissible during fasting. While we tend to normally think of breaking a fast in terms of succumbing to the temptation to eat a large hamburger and some ice cream, there are subtle ways of accidentally breaking your fast that you should studiously avoid. Supplements such as gummy multivitamins, for example, can contain enough sugar, fat and protein to break your fast. Likewise, Branched-chain amino acids (BCAAs) can trigger an insulin response that may oppose the healthy autophagy partially responsible for conferring the benefits of fasting discussed earlier. Protein powder likewise contains enough calories to trigger an insulin response, which can impede the metabolic switching response which contributes to the benefits of fasting. In general, anything containing ingredients like cane sugar, fruit juice concentrates, calories, pectin or maltodextrin can break your fast prematurely and ought to be avoided.

On the other hand, probiotics and prebiotics contain no calories or digestible carbohydrates and are therefore permissible. Pure collagen might slightly impede autophagy but should not significantly affect your fast. Multivitamins, provided they do not contain either sugar or added fillers, contain so few calories (if any) that they should not be a problem. Individual micronutrients such as Vitamin D, B vitamins or potassium are permissible. Fat-soluble vitamins, however, which does include vitamin D (and also A, E, and K) are best absorbed when taken with food. Creatine is likewise permissible as it is calorie-free and does not trigger an insulin response.

# Fasting with Friends

Fasting does not have to be a solemn activity that is done in isolation as a reclusive hermit. Instead, it is something that you can practice with sympathetic friends who may have similar goals as your own and may also have similar beliefs associated with your own. The benefits that may accrue from the social elements of fasting are obvious when they take place within a religious context. For example, if you are a Buddhist monk, you may spend a great deal of your time fasting with your fellow monks in the Sangha (Buddhist community). Of course, you may do this as a Buddhist even if you are not a monk. Likewise, if you are a Muslim, you may enjoy attending Mosque during Ramadan and discussing spiritual matters among your co-religionists.

Fasting with friends may also be helpful due to the benefit of mutual accountability and sympathetic sharing of the struggles of fasting. You do not, for example, have to struggle in silence with respect to your hunger pains, and talking with your friends about your struggles may help alleviate them and distract you from them without causing you to feel strange if you were to share these concerns with others who do not engage in fasting.

## Fasting and Cardio

Although not necessarily restricted to the practice of intermittent fasting, the concept of "fasted cardio" is quickly becoming a hot topic within the fitness world. To be sure, you will often find yourself on either an empty or a near-empty stomach while fasting, and it is permissible to exercise during this time as long as it is done safely. The underlying rationale for attempting this is due to the tendency of fasted cardio to burning larger amounts of fat. Because you do not possess excess calories from a recent meal that your body can rely upon as stored fuel, your body resorts to burning both stored fat and glycogen. Some studies even suggest that working out in the morning after 8-12 hours of fasting during sleep may allow you to burn up to 20 percent more fat, although research on this is inconclusive (Weatherspoon, 2018).

Nevertheless, it is important to be clear about what you are trying to accomplish with your workout before attempting fasted cardio. If you are using your workout to try to build muscle, fasted cardio may be counterproductive as you may end up losing muscle mass. However, if the particular intermittent fasting protocol you are following does not require total abstinence from food, your muscle mass should be well-protected as long as you are consistently consuming protein, as you ought to be doing during fasting protocols that do not require total food abstinence anyway (Weatherspoon, 2018). You may find it helpful to time your workout strategically relative to your fasting protocol, in such a way that allows you to eat after exercising, so that any muscle breakdown that occurred during the workdown can be repaired. Ideally, it is recommended that you consume about 20 grams of protein within 30 minutes after your workout if you are engaging in strength training.

Of course, some people simply enjoy the experience of working out on an empty stomach. This is not necessarily surprising, since exercising and fasting are both associated with endorphin release. In fact, some research suggests that one of the causal mechanisms that may mediate the antidepressant effect of fasting may be precisely this mood-lifting secretion of one of the brain's favorite endogenous peptides.

Whatever your preference, it is certainly better to engage in intense workout on an empty stomach than on a very full stomach. Eating too much prior to intense cardio may cause serious gastrointestinal distress and ought to be avoided. Foods that are high in fat and high in fiber are especially to be avoided, and the negative impact of exercising intensely on an empty stomach can be even more serious in the morning. If you have eaten a sizable portion, it is important to allow at least two hours of digestion before attempting any serious cardio. Other than that, a light but healthy snack is a good precursor to working out and working out on an empty stomach should pose no problems either, as long as you are sufficiently hydrated and are not engaging in an unusually extreme fast. Keep in mind that it may not be wise to work out on an empty stomach, however, if you are about to perform an activity that requires an unusually high level of either speed or power. Since the sort of glucose your body prefers specifically for activities involving very high levels of speed and power will be in short supply, exercising on an empty stomach is something you should only do if you are simply engaging in an ordinary, healthy workout routine rather than running a marathon.

Cardio on an empty stomach is definitely not for everyone, and those with certain health conditions may experience dizziness during such activities. This may lead to increased risk of injury from low blood sugar or low blood pressure. Aside from the fact that these states can be inherently dangerous, the last thing you want to do while running is pass out and end up in a face plant on the road! Such cardio workouts, done on an empty stomach, should be of moderate intensity at most and should not exceed 60 minutes without any food consumption (Weatherspoon, 2018). As always, be sure to stay hydrated. Finally, make sure to listen to your body and never do anything that produces severe discomfort. Those with any health conditions or concerns about fasted cardio ought to consult a physician.

Although those with diabetes or metabolic syndrome ought to be careful while fasting, and should consult with a doctor prior to beginning to fast, some research suggests that exercising while fasting affects muscle biochemistry linked with both blood sugar levels and insulin sensitivity in a way that might be particularly risky for those with these conditions. Individuals with such conditions who are fasting may therefore want to eat and then immediately exercise prior to the onset of digestion or absorption.

Some research shows that exercising while fasting affects muscle biochemistry and metabolism that's linked to insulin sensitivity and the steady control of blood sugar levels. Research also supports eating and immediately exercising before digestion or absorption occurs. This is particularly important for anyone with type 2 diabetes or metabolic syndrome. Some researchers insist that combining intense exercise with intermittent fasting is less than ideal because it depletes the body of its calories and energy which could actually slow your metabolism, defeating the purpose of fasting.

Of course, your relationship between intermittent fasting and exercise depends a great deal upon which intermittent fasting regimen you are employing, and the manner in which you are exercising within the context of this regimen. For example, we have looked at the 16:8 Leangains protocol, in which you consume all food within an 8-hour window and then fast again for 16 hours. Working out prior to the 8-hour food window might work for someone who can exercise well on an empty stomach. However, working out during this window might be better for someone who prefers to exercise not long after having eaten and wants to ensure that they maximally utilize their post-exercise nutrition. Some specialists argue that this method is optimal for performance and recovery, although it may be necessary for some of those who are fasting to work out during the period in which they are fasting if their schedule necessitates it.

How you ought to optimally manage your exercise routine within the context of your fasting regimen also depends in large measure upon the kinds of food you are eating during your consumption window. Strength workouts require larger levels of carbohydrates during the day of the workout routine, while cardio or high-intensity interval training is permissible when lower levels of carbohydrates are consumed.

## The Benefits of Coffee While Fasting

Since a cup of black coffee contains only 3 calories and tiny amounts of fat, protein and trace minerals, it is not likely to break your fast (Hill, 2019). Even two cups are not usually enough to produce a sufficiently major metabolic change of the sort that would break a fast. It is important, however, to not add any ingredients, since this may increase the number of calories, and therefore, the likelihood of impeding the desired metabolic shift responsible for fasting's desired impact. Adding high-calorie ingredients like milk and sugar can be particularly disruptive to your intermittent fasting routine, and you should therefore avoid certain Starbucks drinks you may otherwise enjoy. Intriguingly, black coffee may enhance the benefits of fasting due to its tendency to suppress appetite. It may also reduce blood sugar and its associated risk of type 2 diabetes, reduce inflammation and decrease heart disease risk and risk of metabolic syndrome. In fact, up to 3 cups of black coffee a day is associated with a nearly 20 percent reduced risk of death from heart disease (Hill, 2019).

Just as intermittent fasting itself may improve brain health and reduce risks associated with neurological problems, research suggests that coffee itself may protect against both Alzheimer's and Parkinson's disease. In fact, just as fasting has been found to produce energy from fat in the form of ketones, which is associated with improved brain function, some research suggests that caffeine may likewise promote ketone production and augment this effect of fasting. Intermittent fasting and coffee alike both appear to significantly enhance autophagy, sought after among those practicing intermittent fasting due to its health benefits (Hill, 2019).

As with anything, coffee intake should be conducted in moderation, especially for those engaged in intermittent fasting, as some of the side effects of excess caffeine consumption can offset the advantages of fasting. Drinking up to 13 cups a day can result in increased fasting insulin levels, leading to decreased insulin sensitivity. Too much coffee can also negatively impact your sleep quality, leading to metabolic health problems, which can interfere with the benefits of fasting. Generally speaking, 3-4 cups of coffee a day has been shown to be safe for most people, although you should reduce your intake or cease altogether if you find that you begin to have heart palpitations (Hill, 2019).

# Gender Differences in Fasting

As is the case with many health-related issues, fasting does not affect men and women in the same way. Although properly conducted fasting is safe and healthy for men and women, it does not appear to be as beneficial for women as it is for men, and for this reason, it must be conducted with special caution among women. One study actually found that blood sugar levels worsened in women after three weeks of intermittent fasting, which did not occur among the men. Because women are especially sensitive to calorie restriction, they are more likely to experience changes in their menstrual cycles after beginning one of these protocols (Coyle, 2018).

Frequent or prolonged low caloric intake in women can impact a part of the brain called the hypothalamus in a way that disrupts secretion of gonadotropin-releasing hormone (GnRH), which assists in the release of luteinizing hormone (LH) and follicle stimulating hormone (FSH). Such a disruption can interfere with the ability of these hormones to communicate with the ovaries, leading to irregular periods, problems with bone health, infertility and other harmful effects. In fact, studies on female rats have shown that 3-6 months of alternate day fasting resulted in a reduction in ovary size and abnormal reproductive cycles. Nevertheless, it should be noted that no comparable human studies have been conducted (Coyle, 2018).

This does not, however, mean that women cannot or ought not fast. Instead, it may simply be necessary to modify the means by which they engage in intermittent fasting. This can include fewer fasting days or shorter fasting periods or a combination of both. Despite the risks that can sometimes be associated with intermittent fasting among women, one study has found that obese women who practiced intermittent fasting lowered blood pressure by 6 percent in only eight weeks and also found that this practice lowered LDL cholesterol by 25 percent and triglycerides by 32 percent. Another study of over 100 overweight or obese women who engaged in intermittent fasting for 6 months exhibited reduced insulin levels by almost 30 percent and insulin resistance by almost 20 percent, although blood sugar levels remained the same (Coyle, 2018).

Although there is no universally suitable method of intermittent fasting for women, there are some protocols that tend to be more suitable for women than others. One form of fasting is known as the crescendo method, which involves fasting 12-16 hours for between two and three non-consecutive days a week. Many of the other intermittent fasting protocols that we have discussed are safe and effective for women. Although the eat-stop-eat protocol, also known as the 24-hour protocol, which entails a full 24-hour fast once or twice a week, is safe for women, it may be more appropriate to begin with 14-16-hour fasts. The 5:2 Diet, modified alternate day fasting and the 16/8 method, all of which have been discussed earlier, are all recommended for women. As always, of course, women who are pregnant or are trying to conceive, have fertility problems or a history of amenorrhea or who begin to experience problems such as loss of their menstrual cycle, should not engage in fasting and should consult a physician.

## Combining Intermittent Fasting with Keto

Despite the popularity of the helpful keto diet, whose purpose is to help your body reach a state in which it is burning ketones in such a way that contributes to weight loss, it is not always an adequate means of reaching ketosis in isolation. For those who struggle in reaching this end, intermittent fasting may actually help your body reach this state more quickly and smoothly than the keto diet. However, it may actually be beneficial to combine both protocols in order to maximize intended results.

The underlying purpose of the ketogenic (keto) diet is to eat high levels of fat but low levels of carbohydrates, typically under 50 grams per day. This forces your body to rely on fats as its primary energy supply rather than glucose. The reader may recall that during the much sought after metabolic shift experienced in properly conducted intermittent fasting, the body begins to rely on ketones for its alternate energy source, as a product of having evolved to endure periods of famine. This diet has been found to have a large number of health benefits, many of which overlap with the benefits of intermittent fasting. These benefits include improving symptoms associated with Alzheimer's disease, enhanced insulin resistance, lowered risk of heart disease and reduced blood sugar.

In both intermittent fasting and the keto diet, you are trying to put your body into the metabolic state known as ketosis. Instead of putting your body into this state through flipping the metabolic switch by means of intermittent fasting, the keto diet attempts to reach this state by dramatically reducing carbohydrate intake and replacing it with fat. This, as we have seen, causes the body to very efficiently burn fat as a source of energy by converting fat into ketones within the liver. The ketogenic diet has also been shown to cause huge reductions in insulin levels and blood sugar and when combined with use of ketones as a source of energy, tremendous health benefits have been shown to accrue.

As within intermittent fasting, the ketogenic diet refers to a broad class of food consumption protocols rather than a single isolated method. For example, while the cyclical ketogenic diet involves periods of higher-carbohydrate refeeds, such as 5 ketogenic days followed by 2 high-carbohydrate days, the standard ketogenic diet is a very low-carbohydrate and high-fat diet that contains 75 percent fat, 20 percent protein and only 4 percent carbohydrates. The targeted ketogenic diet allows you to add carbohydrates around workouts while the high-protein ketogenic diet includes more protein and less fat. Generally speaking, most people who practice one of the ketogenic protocols follow either the standard or high-protein ketogenic diets, both of which are the only variants of this regimen that have been studied extensively.

Ketogenic protocols have been extensively studied and consistently found to yield impressive health benefits. One study found that those on the ketogenic diet lost 3 times more weight than those on a regimen recommended by Diabetes UK. Yet another study found that those on a ketogenic diet lost 2.2 times more weight than those on a calorie-restricted diet whose purpose is to decrease fat, also resulting in healthier triglyceride and HDL cholesterol levels (Mawer, 2018). Indeed, these protocols are very effective at helping you lose the excess fat that is closely linked with serious health problems like metabolic syndrome, prediabetes and type 2 diabetes. In fact, one study found that the ketogenic diet can improve insulin sensitivity by an incredible 75 percent (Mawer). These effects are so dramatic that research has found that as much as a third of diabetic participants were able to stop using diabetes medications altogether.

Those participating in the ketogenic diet should avoid sugary foods, fruit, grains, starches, beans, legumes, tubers, root vegetables, low-fat and diet products, unhealthy fats, alcohol and sugar-free foods. Instead, they should stick with meat, butter, cream, eggs, cheese, nuts and seeds, healthy oils, avocados, condiments and low-carbohydrate veggies. Some individuals may physically struggle with the ketogenic diet due to a set of side effects known as "keto flu." Although uncomfortable, these side effects usually subside within a few days and include sleep issues, nausea, decreased exercise performance, digestive problems, hunger and lower energy. These symptoms can be mitigated by trying an ordinary low-carbohydrate diet for the first few weeks before going full-keto right away, allowing your body to become accustomed to burning more fat prior to totally eliminating all carbohydrates. Since this diet can alter your body's water and mineral balance, taking mineral supplements or adding salt to your meals can help.

Many of those attempting the keto diet have struggled effectively reaching ketosis but combining one of these protocols with intermittent fasting may assist in this process. This can be quite challenging, however, as many of those who combine both may have a hard time resisting the temptation to overeat on non-fasting days and may find themselves beset with fatigue and irritability. Therefore, although combining a ketogenic protocol with intermittent fasting may be helpful, the difficulty involved may not be optimal for everyone.

Those who are attempting to enter into ketosis, whether through intermittent fasting or one of the ketogenic diet protocols or a combination of both, may find it helpful to begin to include coconut oil in their diets. Coconut oil contains fats known as medium-chain triglycerides (MCTs) which, unlike most fats, are quickly absorbed into the liver where they can immediately be used for energy or converted into ketones. About 50 percent of the MCT fat from coconut oil comes from a substance known as lauric acid. Research suggests that far sources with a higher percentage of this substance may contribute to more sustained levels of ketosis due to how gradually it is metabolized relative to other MCTs.

Some sources even suggest that consuming coconut oil may be one of the most effective ways of increasing ketone levels in people with nervous system disorders such as Alzheimer's disease. Astonishingly, some research has suggested that MCTs are so powerful that they can induce ketosis without restricting carbs as dramatically as those who participate in the classic ketogenic diet. Several studies have found that a diet high in MCTs, containing 20 percent of calories from carbs, produces effects similar to the classic ketogenic diet, and this has allowed these substances to induce ketosis in epileptic children without restricting carbohydrates to the same degree as those who use one of the keto protocols (O'Brien, 2018).

While these specialized fats are particularly conducive to reaching a state of ketosis, consuming a lot of healthy fat in general is effective in boosting your ketone levels to a degree that will help you reach ketosis. This is why ketogenic diets are not only low in carbohydrates, but high in fat. Generally speaking, these protocols recommend that you acquire 60-80 percent of your calories from healthy fat sources. These fat sources ought to include, not only coconut oil, but avocado oil, lard, butter and tallow.

Testing your ketone levels may help in determining whether your particular protocol and habits are effectively moving you towards your goal. Since what moves one particular individual to ketosis may differ substantially from what gets it done for another, those engaged in intermittent fasting or a ketogenic protocol or a combination of both are encouraged to undergo tests that measure three forms of ketones detectable in breath, urine and blood. These substances are acetone, beta-hydroxybutyrate and acetoacetate. Acetone is present in your breath and research has confirmed that using the proper instruments to measure acetone breath levels is a reliable way to determine whether you are in a state of ketosis among those following ketogenic protocols. It is possible to measure blood ketone levels with only a small drop of blood placed on a strip that is then inserted into a meter.

For those who might be somewhat squeamish when it comes to blood, and who are unwilling to cough up the large amounts of money required for this expensive beta-hydroxybutyrate measurement procedure, the Ketonix meter effectively measures the levels of acetone in your breath and flashes a color that indicates whether you are in a state of ketosis based on the levels of acetone. Finally, ketone urine strips can be dipped into urine and turn various colors, each of which indicate the level of ketones present, with darker ones reflecting higher ketone levels and lighter ones reflecting lower ones. These are much cheaper than the blood tests although not as accurate. Nevertheless, they are generally effective in confirming, at the very least, that you are indeed in a state of ketosis.

## Ketosis and Fat Fasting

Related to the methods employed in the ketogenic protocols, and relevant to those engaged in intermittent fasting who are concerned about what they should be eating during their non-fasting days, is the concept of fat fasting. Like intermittent fasting and the keto diets, the purpose of fat fasting is to raise blood levels of ketones by pushing the body into ketosis in a way that mimics the biological impact of fasting. Of course, this method can be employed within the context of intermittent fasting itself, since it is simply a kind of menu detailing the kinds of foods that are optimal for inducing ketosis and those that may impede the reaction. Those who use this method often claim that, in addition to its positive health effects, it is also an effective means of avoiding or minimizing hunger or food craving while in the midst of fasting.

Although we might tend to intuitively associate a "high fat" diet with an excess of calories, the purpose of fat fasting is actually to produce a caloric deficit in order to cause the body to enter a state in which it relies primarily on ketones for its energy requirements. Perhaps ironically, an appropriate combination of healthy sources of high fat with low levels of carbohydrates will actually help you to burn fat. Importantly, much of the weight lost may reappear if you begin eating carbohydrates again, because it replaces your body's glycogen. Furthermore, loss of carbohydrates also leads to a loss of water which is stored along with glycogen in the form of glucose, which means that much of the weight that you lose can be understood in terms of lost water weight rather than authentic fat loss.

Although high-fat diets (provided the fat is from healthy sources) can be helpful within the context of intermittent fasting, strictly speaking, a fat fast is a fast that is high in fat but low in calories that ordinarily lasts around 2-5 days and allows between 1,000 and 1,200 calories a day, 80 to 90 percent of which ought to come from fat (West,

2019). The purpose of such a regimen is to mimic the effects which authentic fasting has on the human body, namely, putting it into a state of ketosis. As always, mileage may vary, but those who are consistently following a strictly ketogenic diet can expect a state of ketosis at between days 2 and 6 (West, 2019). Even if you have already achieved ketosis, such a diet can be useful because it boosts ketone levels. Even those who are already on a ketogenic diet sometimes adopt this approach if they have hit a kind of plateau and are having trouble losing more weight than they already have. This approach can also be useful for those who have undergone a cheat day and want to recover from any setbacks they may have endured from eating too much.

One method of bursting through one of these troubling plateaus is the so-called egg fast diet, articulated by blogger Jimmy Moore. As the name of the protocol implies, this is a method of fasting whose focus is on obtaining high levels of fat, moderate levels of protein and low levels of carbohydrates from eggs. The fast typically lasts between 3-5 days and its purpose is to enter into a state of ketosis prior to entering into another fasting protocol. Although the original articulation of the diet is fairly strict, it is perfectly permissible for the individual to modify it according to their own needs or desires as long as the general principles of high fat / moderate protein / low carbohydrates are adhered to. In general, this method recommends whole eggs (yolks and whites alike) be the main source of fat and protein, along with 1 tablespoon of butter or healthy fat per egg. In addition to various vitamins and minerals, eggs contain powerful antioxidants that protect eyesight and choline, which contributes to brain health. Disturbingly, research shows that 90 percent of individuals do not consume enough choline (Raman, 2019).

One ounce of full-fat cheese per egg consumed is recommended, and the faster should eat at least six whole eggs per day, preferably local and pastured. Egg consumption ought to begin within 30 minutes of waking up and from then on, an egg-based meal is recommended every 3-5 hours, with food consumption ceasing 3 hours before bedtime. After 3-5 days, whatever weight loss plateau you have encountered should have been overcome (Raman, 2019). Adhering to this protocol for longer than this is not recommended due to health problems that may result, and those with certain chronic conditions such as diabetes and cholesterol hyper-responders, as well as those who lack a gallbladder, should avoid this regimen altogether. Due to the short length of this protocol, it is not best used in isolation, but as a supplementary preface to another form of fasting. Although this method has not been scientifically tested, one of its experiential and widely reported benefits is its tendency to make the individual feel very full, mitigating the hunger that often makes fasting difficult.

This is the product of the high protein content of eggs, which increases hormones that cause a feeling of fullness and prevent the sort of overeating that would eliminate the benefits of fasting. Furthermore, the strict egg-based diet of this regimen sufficiently restricts what you are allowed to eat in a way that will reduce overall caloric intake (Raman, 2019). Apart from these benefits, one of the more obvious benefits of this temporary protocol is that eggs are one of the most nutritious foods on the entire planet (found primarily in the yolk). Furthermore, although whole eggs used to be considered unhealthy in the "old era" due to their high cholesterol and fat, new research suggests that the cholesterol (about 70 percent per egg) in eggs actually does not affect the cholesterol in blood.

While I am not aware of any strict avocado fast, this delicious fruit is another example of a food that is high in healthy fat and perfect for those looking to push their bodies towards ketosis regardless of the protocol they are adhering to. What makes avocados particularly unique is the fact that unlike most fruits, which contain a lot of carbohydrates, avocados have tons of fat. As bizarre as it may sound, avocados consist of almost 80 percent fat by calories, making them higher in fat than even most animal foods. The primary fatty acid is a monounsaturated fat known as oleic acid, which is also found in abundance in olive oil. Avocados also contain a great deal of potassium, even higher levels than that of bananas, and can also lower LDL cholesterol, fiber and triglycerides. Fat itself is not the enemy, and this especially fatty fruit is actually associated with lower levels of belly fat compared to those who do not and have also been shown to have cardiovascular benefits.

An essential component of the Mediterranean diet, extra virgin olive oil contains vitamins E and K, in addition to many powerful antioxidants, which protect against inflammation and LDL particles. This substance is great at improving cardiovascular health, including lower blood pressure, improved cholesterol markers and many other benefits that reduce heart disease risk.

Cheese, a very healthy, low-carbohydrate food that also contains high levels of healthy fats, is especially useful when it comes to dieting. Cheese contains a great deal of protein, phosphorus, selenium, calcium and vitamin B12 as well as other nutrients such as powerful fatty acids that can reduce the risk of type 2 diabetes. Some even undergo a 3-day cottage cheese diet as a means of restricting both carbohydrate and calorie intake. Such a diet, of course, can become quite dull rather quickly and may benefit from various seasoning or spices such as pepper, ginger, Indian spice blends, nutmeg and cinnamon. Nevertheless, adhering to such a protocol may lead to unhealthily high levels of sodium and inadequate nutrition when it comes to the nutrients cheese lacks.

Fatty fish such as trout, salmon, mackerel, herring and sardines are rich in omega-3 fatty acids, proteins and many other nutrients. Like the practice of intermittent fasting in general, these kinds of fish contribute a great deal to both heart and brain health, protecting against depression, dementia and heart disease. In general, consumption of these kinds of fish during fasting is one of the best additions to your regimen. Much good can be said of fatty fish and very little that is bad.

Nuts contain a great deal of healthy fats and fiber, and contain a great deal of protein, providing both the fat needed to burn off unwanted weight and the protein that can prevent the kind of hunger that can tempt you to break your fast through overeating. In fact, almonds, macadamia nuts and walnuts are some of the best sources of plant-based protein available. Nuts contain a great deal of vitamin E and also magnesium, which most people do not consume enough of.

Chia seeds are another example of a food rich in healthy fat and low in carbohydrates. In fact, most of the calories of this food come from fat, at a whopping 80 percent. What's more, the fats in chia seeds are comprised of primarily of the omega-3 fatty acid known as ALA. This morsel lowers blood pressure, and, in addition to the practice of fasting itself, has been shown to lower inflammation.

## The Danger of Diarrhea

Those who experience diarrhea during a fast should cease until their gastrointestinal problems have ceased. Failure to do so may result in nausea, dehydration, malabsorption, malnutrition and dizziness. Since dizziness in particular may already result from intermittent fasting, especially if not conducted properly, diarrhea will only compound these issues to a degree that can become dangerous. It is also important to end your fast if you begin to experience loss of consciousness, chest or abdominal pain and nausea or vomiting. Although diarrhea does not generally result from fasting alone, it can occur during fasting as a result of an over secretion of water and salts in the gastrointestinal tracts. Liquids high in caffeine such as tea or coffee can contribute to this effect. Poor diet, mineral deficiencies, gastrointestinal diseases such as Crohn's disease or ulcerative colitis, infection, food or medication allergy or poor diet may also contribute to the risk of diarrhea (Sethi, 2019).

It is also important to anticipate the possibility that you will experience diarrhea after breaking your fast, since the ability of your bowel to function properly diminishes when it is not used. In order to decrease the chances of this happening, it may be helpful to use the BRAT diet (banana, rice, applesauce, toast). Other foods in this protocol include apple juice, flat soda, broth, boiled potatoes, weak tea, cooked cereals or crackers (Butler, 2019). Avoid any dairy products, anything fried, greasy, spicy or fatty, drinks that are either very hot or very cold or which contain alcohol or caffeine, raw veggies or foods with high levels of protein. Of course, it is permissible to eat at least some of these foods when breaking your fast, and these recommendations are relevant primarily for those who may struggle with diarrhea after breaking their fast. This involves eating food that is bland, starchy and low in fiber, because such a consumption protocol will replace nutrients and ensure that stool remains firm. Fried food, beans and broccoli may also increase the risk of diarrhea, so it is advised to avoid such foods when breaking your fast.

Although diarrhea by itself is not typically dangerous, you should consult a doctor immediately if you begin to experience pain during bowel movements, bloody stool or swelling around the bowel. Since diarrhea can interfere with your fast and cause you to break it, it is important to do what you can to prevent it from occurring. Drinking lots of water, diluted juice, weak tea, and electrolyte-replacement drinks like Gatorade can help. Avoid other sugary drinks, especially those with caffeine, and make sure to consume food that is high in soluble fiber, potassium and salt.

# Intermittent Fasting and Sex Drive

Importantly for some people, intermittent fasting may interfere negatively with your sex drive, partially as a product of its tendency to lower the amount of energy you have for physical activity, and associated irritability and lightheadedness. Exactly what your diet consists of, however, largely determines whether or to what extent your sex drive will be adversely impacted. Those who are consuming foods high in protein, healthy fat and vitamins during non-fasting periods may experience a relatively normal and healthy sex drive, whereas those who suffer from a deficit in these areas (either as a product of fasting or for other reasons) may have a lower sex drive. Those who struggle with fasting and end up succumbing to the temptation to break their fast or compromise it in other ways may likewise feel guilt or shame that may lower their sex drive as well (Hendricks, 2018).

One study on the impact of erectile function and sexual desire on men during the month of Ramadan found that the fasting associated with this duration may be associated with lower levels of sexual desire and serum FSH levels. Participants in this study were asked to complete two domains of International Index of Erectile Function (IIEF) questionnaire for erectile function and sexual desire and also to provide information on smoking habits, frequency of sexual intercourse, any diseases, or any treatment they were undergoing for those who had been diagnosed with a disease. By the end of the month, serum follicle stimulating hormones had decreased significantly relative to their baseline levels, but no significant impact was found with respect to either erectile function or testosterone. Nevertheless, such intermittent fasting protocols may be associated with lower levels of sexual desire and lower frequency of sexual intercourse (Talib et. al).

# Resources

Anton, Stephen D., Moehl, Keelin, Donahoo, William T., Marosi, Krizstina, Lee, Stephanie, Mainous, Arch G., Leeuwenburgh, Christiaan, Mattson, Mark P (2018, April 30). Flipping the Metabolic Switch: Understanding and Applying Health Benefits of Fasting. *Obesity (Silver Spring). 2018 Feb; 26*(2): 254–268. doi: 10.1002/oby.22065

Berger, Matt (2019, August 22). How Intermittent Fasting Can Help Lower Inflammation. Retrieved from: https://www.healthline.com/health-news/fasting-can-help-ease-inflammation-in-the-body#Diet-and-inflammation

Bjarnadottir, Adda (2020, February 25th). Alternate-Day Fasting: A Comprehensive Beginner's Guide. Retrieved from: https://www.healthline.com/nutrition/alternate-day-fasting-guide

Butler, Natalie (2019, March 7). BRAT Diet: What Is It and Does It Work?

Retrieved from: https://www.healthline.com/health/brat-diet#:~:text=You%20can%20eat%20more%20than,by%20firming%20up%20your%20stools.

Butler, Natalie (2019, October 30). Everything You Want to Know About Dry Fasting. Retrieved from: https://www.healthline.com/health/food-nutrition/dry-fasting#purported-benefits

Coyle, Daisy (2018, July 22). Intermittent Fasting For Women: A Beginner's Guide. Retrieved from: https://www.healthline.com/nutrition/intermittent-fasting-for-women

Gaikwad, Sandip T (2017). Apprehending Concept, Canons and Types of

Fasting in Buddhism. National Institute of Food Technology Entrepreneurship and Management. Volume 2, Issue 4. Retrieved from: http://www.ijirct.org/papers/IJIRCT1601028.pdf

Giovannelli, Gloriane. How to Not Sabotage Yourself while Fasting. Retrieved from: https://drgloriane.com/stop-self-sabotage-while-fasting/

Gunnars, Kris (2020, January 1). 6 Popular Ways to Do Intermittent Fasting. Retrieved from: https://www.healthline.com/nutrition/6-ways-to-do-intermittent-fasting

Hebebrand, Johannes, Albayrak, Özgür, Adan, Roger, Antel, Joche, Dieguez, Carlos, de Jong, Jjohannes, Leng, Gareth, Menzies, ohn, Mercer, Julian, Murphy, Michelle, van der Plasse, Geoffrey, Dickson, Suzanne L. (2014 November). "Eating addiction", rather than "food addiction", better captures addictive-like eating behavior. *Neuroscience & Biobehavioral Reviews Volume 47, November 2014,* Pages 295-306. https://doi.org/10.1016/j.neubiorev.2014.08.016

Hendricks, Sara (2018, August 28). Intermittent fasting could diminish your sex drive — but there's a way to revive it. Retrieved from: https://www.insider.com/how-does-intermittent-fasting-diet-affect-sex-drive-2018-8

Henriques, Carolina (2016, December 16). Fasting May Help to Prevent Seizures by Calming Nervous System, Early Study Suggests. Retrieved from: https://epilepsynewstoday.com/2016/12/16/fasting-may-reduce-epileptic-seizures-by-calming-nervous-system/

Hill, Ansley (2019, June 14). Can You Drink Coffee While Doing Intermittent Fasting?

 Retrieved from:
https://www.healthline.com/nutrition/intermittent-fasting-coffee#basics

Hindu fasting in the workplace: An awareness guide for staff and managers (2019). Retrieved from:
https://civilservice.blog.gov.uk/wp-content/uploads/sites/86/2019/10/hindu-fasting-in-the-workplace-awareness-guide-1.pdf

Intermittent fasting: A "new" historical strategy for controlling seizures?

Adam L. Hartman, James E. Rubenstein, Eric H. Kossoff

Epilepsy Res. Author manuscript; available in PMC 2014 May 1.

Published in final edited form as: Epilepsy Res. 2013 May; 104(3): 275–279. Published online 2012 Dec 1. doi: 10.1016/j.eplepsyres.2012.10.011

PMCID: PMC3740951

Jauregui, Ruth de (2016, Jan. 16). NIH study identifies protein that may prevent obesity-related inflammation. Retrieved from:
https://patientdaily.com/stories/510658262-nih-study-identifies-protein-that-may-prevent-obesity-related-inflammation

Kubala, Jillian (2019, December 1). 23 Simple Things You Can Do to Stop Overeating. Retrieved from:
https://www.healthline.com/nutrition/how-to-stop-overeating#section3

Marengo, Katherine (2020, February 25). Intermittent Fasting for Psoriasis: Is It Safe and Can It Help? Retrieved from: https://www.healthline.com/health/psoriasis/fasting-for-psoriasis

Mawer, Rudy (2018, July 30). The Ketogenic Diet: A Detailed Beginner's Guide to Keto. Retrieved from: https://www.healthline.com/nutrition/ketogenic-diet-101

O'Brien, Sharon (2018, May 14). 7 Science-Based Benefits of MCT Oil. Retrieved from: https://www.healthline.com/nutrition/mct-oil-benefits#section3

Olsen, Natalie (2020, January 6). Everything You Should Know About Refeeding Syndrome. Retrieved from: https://www.healthline.com/health/refeeding-syndrome

Preiato, Daniel (2019, May 23). Everything You Need to Know About 48-Hour Fasting. Retrieved from: https://www.healthline.com/nutrition/48-hour-fasting

Raman, Ryan How to Do an Egg Fast: Rules, Benefits, and Sample Menu. (2019, February 28). Retrieved from: https://www.healthline.com/nutrition/egg-fast

Raman, Ryan (2019, December 17). Water Fasting: Benefits and Dangers. Retrieved from: https://www.healthline.com/nutrition/water-fasting

Ramos, Megan (2020 March 19). How to Break Your Fast: https://www.dietdoctor.com/intermittent-fasting/how-to-break-your-fast

References: Fasting-Mimicking Diet Modulates Microbiota and Promotes Intestinal Regeneration to Reduce Inflammatory Bowel Disease Pathology. Rangan P, Choi I, Wei M, Navarrete G, Guen E, Brandhorst S, Enyati N, Pasia G, Maesincee D, Ocon V, Abdulridha

M, Longo VD. Cell Rep. 2019 Mar 5;26(10):2704-2719.e6. doi: 10.1016/j.celrep.2019.02.019. PMID: 30840892.

Sethi, Saurabh (2019, October 7). Diarrhea During Fasting and Other Side Effects. Retrieved from: https://www.healthline.com/health/diarrhea-during-fasting

Talib RA, Canguven O, Al-Rumaihi K, Al Ansari A, Alani M. The effect of fasting on erectile function and sexual desire on men in the month of Ramadan. Urol J. 2015;12(2):2099-2102. Published 2015 Apr 29.

Weatherspoon, Deborah (2018, September 11). Can You Lose Weight Faster by Exercising on an Empty Stomach? Retrieved from: https://www.healthline.com/health/fitness-exercise/fasted-cardio-when-to-eat-workout#6

West, Helen (2019, April 29). What Is Fat Fasting, and Is It Good for You? Retrieved from: https://www.healthline.com/nutrition/keto-fat-fast

Zelman, Kathleen M (2019, May 9). What to Do After You Overeat. Retrieved from: https://www.webmd.com/diet/ss/slideshow-what-to-do-after-overeating

Zhang, Yifan, Liu, Changhong, Zhao, Yinghao, Zhang, Xingyi, Li, Bingjin, Cui, Ranji (2015 July). The Effects of Calorie Restriction in Depression and Potential Mechanisms. *Curr Neuropharmacol. 2015 Jul; 13*(4): 536–542. doi: 10.2174/1570159X13666150326003852